Mosby's
Biomedical Science Series

UNDERSTANDING
Epidemiology

Mosby's
Biomedical Science Series

UNDERSTANDING
Epidemiology

MARY E. TORRENCE, DVM, Ph.D., Dipl. ACVPM
Epidemiologist and Team Leader
Epidemiology Team
Office of Surveillance and Biometrics
Center for Devices and Radiological Health
Food and Drug Administration
Rockville, Maryland

and

Adjunct Professor
Department of Biomedical Sciences
Virginia-Maryland Regional College of Veterinary Medicine
Virginia Polytechnic Institute and State University
Blacksburg, Virginia

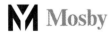 Mosby

St. Louis Baltimore Boston Carlsbad Chicago Naples New York Philadelphia Portland
London Madrid Mexico City Singapore Sydney Tokyo Toronto Wiesbaden

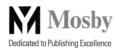

Mosby

Dedicated to Publishing Excellence

A Times Mirror
Company

Vice President and Publisher: Don Ladig
Executive Editor: Paul W. Pratt
Senior Developmental Editor: Teri Merchant
Project Manager: Patricia Tannian
Production Editor: Melissa Mraz Lastarria
Book Design Manager: Gail Morey Hudson
Manufacturing Manager: Dave Graybill
Cover Designer: Teresa Breckwoldt

Printed in the United States of America
Composition by Clarinda Company
Printing/binding by Maple Vail Book Mfg. Group

Mosby–Year Book, Inc.
11830 Westline Industrial Drive
St. Louis, Missouri 63146

Library of Congress Cataloging in Publication Data

Torrence, Mary E.
    Understanding epidemiology/Mary E. Torrence.
        p.   cm.—(Mosby's biomedical science series)
    Includes bibliographical references and index.
    ISBN 0–8151–8887–0
    1. Epidemiology, I. Title. II. Series.
    [DNLM: 1. Epidemiology. WA 105 T691u 1997]
    RA651.T67 1997
    614.4—dc21
    DNLM/DLC   96–39467
    for Library of Congress   CIP

96 97 98 99 00 / 9 8 7 6 5 4 3 2 1

Introduction

"It seems very pretty," she said when she had finished it, "but it's rather hard to understand!" (You see she didn't like to confess, even to herself, that she couldn't make it out at all.) "Somehow it seems to fill my head with ideas—only I don't exactly know what they are!"

-Lewis Carroll, *Through the Looking Glass*

When I came across this quote while reading James Schlesselman's dissent on the selection of case-control studies (*J. Chron. Dis.* 38:549-550, 1985), I thought it was an appropriate description for both the discipline of epidemiology and the writing process of this book. Epidemiology is a field of science that is complex at first glimpse, but once understood gives a logical, systematic approach to understanding the complexities of disease. Epidemiology is an ever-expanding discipline that offers its methodology and concepts for the use in other scientific endeavors.

When medical and veterinary medical students are first introduced to epidemiology, the subject appears difficult and confusing. This is not because of the complexity or difficulty of the subject but rather the fact that epidemiology requires reasoning. Epidemiology is not the memorization of facts but rather the art and the ability of thinking—critical and insightful thinking. This can be daunting territory. Epidemiology instills the thought process, the methodology, and the techniques to approach a problem and the ability to pursue its answer. I guess that is why epidemiologists are often called "medical detectives." This field is a wonderful asset to those of us that love to explore all kinds of subjects, problems, and diseases.

Although epidemiologic thinking seems to be an ancient discipline, it is also still in its infancy. Epidemiologic thinking and studies have been traced as far back as Hippocrates, circa 400 BC. One of the past heroes in epidemiology was a London haberdasher named John Graunt who in 1662 first analyzed and described mortality data. He explained patterns of gender differences, urban versus rural differences, and seasonal differences. These same patterns are used today. The father of surveillance is William Farr who in the mid 1800s began to collect Britain's mortality data and to develop vital statistics, as well as methods of disease classification, that are still used today. Finally, the father of field epidemiology is John Snow who conducted a number of investigations in London in 1854 to determine the cause of cholera outbreaks 20 years before the microscope. His work is cited in almost every epidemiologic textbook.

The future of epidemiology looks even brighter with more growth. The expansive world of computer technology has already begun to increase the possibilities for epidemiologic advancement. Computers have allowed quick access to large databases of information that can be searched and analyzed. Hospitals are initiating computer-based patient records that will allow epidemiologists access to medical data. Even the Internet allows greater accessibility to new journal articles, communications with other epidemiologists, and other related information. The field of molecular biology has made giant leaps in knowledge and technology that have and will continue to expand the ability of epidemiologists to track down the causes and risk factors for disease. New laboratory techniques and tests have allowed epidemiologists to trace the sources of various infectious outbreaks.

As a part of Mosby's Biomedical Series, this book is intended to be a short, concise text on the main concepts and principles of epidemiology. It is not meant to be the complete resource for a course. This is a textbook to help students understand the field in such a way to enable them to concentrate on more technical and difficult concepts.

As stated in the beginning quotation, I had many ideas but was uncertain of the direction. After years of studying epidemiology, I still found myself delving into hours of thinking and researching to understand all the complexities. I have always searched for a short, concise, yet understandable principle.

This book is not intended for expert epidemiologists but for those students who are beginning their experiences in the field of epidemiology. It is my hope that this book will aid in the understanding of the main principles and concepts of epidemiology and will allow the student to progress to more difficult, technical concepts.

This book may incite some criticism from my peers for two reasons. One, this text is a limited and shortened look at epidemiology. I could not cover all of the facts or even all of the concepts, though I had to restrain myself at times from trying. I am certain that there will be some of my peers who think I should have covered or emphasized other concepts within epidemiology or that I focused too much on certain other principles. My goal was to cover the principles I felt most important. Two, I am certain that some of the principles I have presented are not universally accepted. The field of epidemiology is full of differences in opinion both in terminology used, as well as in the meaning of some of the concepts. These differences are not resolved and probably will never be. Part of the art of critical thinking is the differences in thought and opinions and the discussions that arise from those differences. From those discussions and reasonings come new ideas and new approaches. Like all scientists, I chose what I believe to be true, but I enjoy the lively discussions of what others see as true. It is my intent for students to be stimulated to think critically about the information presented.

My hope is that this textbook will help provide understanding and insight to the field of epidemiology. My selfish desire is to stimulate curious minds to at least entertain the thought of pursuing epidemiology.

M.E.T.

Series Preface

Science textbooks are commonly entitled "Principles of . . ." Yet almost all of these books go far beyond principles to specify so much detail that they often obscure the principles. Too often the emphasis is on currently accepted facts, with principles used only to illustrate the facts, rather than using the minimum amount of fact to illustrate principles.

This situation argues for a new kind of textbook, one that focuses on the first principles of the discipline. In addition to encyclopedic tomes for each discipline, we need small texts that give the big picture and explicitly describe the basic foundational principles of the discipline—and no more!

As a start to what I hope will be a new movement in science education we are initiating a series of biomedical science teaching books that really are about principles. These books aim to be quick, yet elegant, overviews of the essence of the respective disciplines. The newcomer to the subject should find the preparation needed to understand the more comprehensive and detailed traditional textbooks and research journals. Maybe even highly specialized experts can find some useful perspectives from this approach. Senior people tend to get wrapped up in the details of their specialty and sometimes take the principles for granted.

We must have some kind of working definition of "principle." While many ways can express the idea, this Series of texts uses the following working definition:

> A principle must go beyond a collection of observations. Principles integrate multiple observations and help to explain these observations, providing understanding and insight. A principle embodies the underlying rules or mechanisms of structure, organization, or operation that give rise to the observations. We distinguish principles from concepts only in the sense that concepts often embody more than one principle.

In identifying these principles, we must recognize that they are basic tenets; i.e., commonly held *beliefs* about what is true and fundamental. Not everyone will agree that each of these "principles" deserves such lofty status. However, there is a fine line between principle and theory. Theories serve to inspire better theories that can establish principles more firmly.

Many of the statements of principle are incomplete. They may also lack sufficient qualification. Statements of principles serve to inspire more complete or precise exposition. The effort to identify principles comes at a cost: arbitrariness, uncertainty, controversy—but the cost is worth the price. *The search for principles is the Holy Grail of science.*

The practical value of such texts may lie in their pedagogical approach, which is the opposite from the tack taken in many textbooks on biological and medical subjects. Students are fed up with encyclopedic subjects. Students and professors alike are tired of an educational process devoted to pouring information into one ear while it spills out the other. The exponential expansion of new knowledge is causing cognitive overload in students and professors, short-circuiting their ability to sustain perspective about the whole of biomedical science and to think coherently about the details of how the body works in both health and disease. We are learning more and more about less and less, and that causes a progressive loss of capacity for synthesis and ability to think about the larger meanings of biomedical science. The texts in this series require the student to be actively involved in completing missing detail and providing the qualifications of special relevance.

Why These Books Are Needed

- Traditional texts are too big, too detailed, too indigestible
- Biomedical information is accumulating faster than students can handle
- Students are learning more and more about less and less
- Students, and even teachers, have trouble discerning the "must know" from the "nice to know"
- The new emphasis in teaching of biomedical sciences will be on how to manage, integrate, and apply information. That requires identification and understanding of the basic principles of the discipline.

The advantages of books in this Series, as I see it, are as follows:

Advantages to Students:

- Students more likely to "see the forest instead of the trees"
  - What is important is made explicit
  - Cognitive overload can't obscure perspective and insight
- "Less is More"
  - Less material is easier to comprehend and remember
  - It is easier to remember unifying principles and concepts
  - Understanding principles empowers students to get more from new information
- Promotes active learning, critical thinking, insight, understanding
- Very useful in self-paced or collaborative learning paradigms
  - Helps assure that students have the required background
  - Students are better prepared to understand what they read in journals and reference books—with minimal help from professors
- Books are smaller, cost less, are more portable, and are easier to peruse
- High portability and condensed nature encourage frequent review
- Longer half-life
  - Traditional texts are out of date as soon as printed
  - Principles are "eternal"

Benefits to Professors

- Allows specialized instruction with less fear that basics are being missed
- After mastering principles, students are equally prepared for subsequent instruction
- Enlivens the lecture period. Meaningful discussion and debate facilitated

Benefits to Graduates

- Quick way to review latest concepts, especially in fields in which they have not kept up
- "User-friendly" access to specialties or to especially complex disciplines

As professors increasingly recognize, the proliferation of research literature has made it difficult to decide what is fundamental about their discipline that must be taught to students. The books in this Series aim to help professors identify that core understanding. Even where a professor may disagree with certain statements of principle, the books provide a focus and a stimulus to the professor to refine those statements of principle with which they disagree.

Where professors believe that more factual detail is needed, they can provide it or direct students to it with some reassurance that students still understand the central core of the discipline. Thus, these books can substitute for the standard, fact-filled textbook and give professors the flexibility to use other instructional media, such as computer-assisted instruction, journal articles, and even standard textbooks as reference sources to complement the Mosby's Biomedical Science Series.

Books in this Series would seem especially important for curricula that stress problem- or case-based learning (PBL). In recognition of the cognitive overload problem some medical schools (McMasters, Harvard, Southern Illinois, Bowman Gray, University of New Mexico) have pioneered in converting the traditional lecture-based curriculum to a tutorial, group-based learning format where critical thinking and information management skills are emphasized rather than rote memory. Some veterinary colleges are also making similar curricular changes. This trend will surely grow, because it is aimed at teaching students to *manage* and *integrate* an ever-expanding biomedical data base.

However, many institutions have thoughtfully considered but rejected PBL-type curricula out of fear that students will have huge gaps in their understanding of the core biomedical science disciplines. Books in this Series not only help PBL students to know what the fundamental principles are, but present them in a quick and easily digestible form. Understanding these principles increases the likelihood that PBL students will truly understand what they read in journals and reference books as they try to apply it to the clinical cases or academic problems.

Organization of These Books

The first—and most difficult—part of writing this kind of text is the identification and terse statement of the first principles of a discipline. Then principles are consolidated, if necessary, and grouped into categories to make it easier to organize and remember them.

Each category has an Introduction that states the principles in that category. There is also a "concept map," which is a diagram that shows the interrelationship of the principles in that category. The authors treat each principle as a module that states the principle and identifies its category. Then the principle is explained, including the use of one or more examples, accompanied by one or two diagrams or pictures. Another section defines key terms, and yet another lists other principles that are most directly related. Finally, a reference section lists two or three key references, along with a list of "Citation Classics,"* where possible. At the end of the modules in a given category, a review section presents some open-ended questions for review and debate.

W.R. (Bill) Klemm

Texas A & M University
College Station, Texas

---

*A "Classic" is a highly cited publication (on the order of 500 or more citations) as identified by the *Science Citation Index,* published by ISI Press, Philadelphia. For some of these, there is an associated publication that appeared in the ISI publication *Current Contents* that contains a history that led up to the research that enabled the publication to have such a major impact. In some cases, the author has taken the liberty to list a publication that in his opinion should have been accorded formal "Classic" status.

Acknowledgements

I want to thank Dr. William Klemm, Series Editor, and Dr. Paul Pratt from Mosby for their support and assistance during the process. I am indebted to Dr. Barbara Silverman, Medical Officer and Epidemiologist, Office of Surveillance and Biometrics, Center for Devices and Radiological Health, Food and Drug Administration, for her careful and insightful review of this book. Her perceptive and critical comments encouraged me to rethink many of the principles and to make the revised text clearer. I learned from our friendly and lively discussions. I would like to thank Kay Freeman for her meticulous editing of my proofs. It was most helpful. I am also indebted to Barbara A. White for her final review of the manuscript for grammar, punctuation, and wording. She is a retired English teacher who taught many students, including me, the importance of the writing process. I have the utmost respect for her as a gifted teacher and as a person. I am continually indebted to my family. This textbook, as well as other accomplishments, would not have been achieved without their support, encouragement, and presence.

Organization of the Book

The main principles or concepts in this book are grouped into categories to make them easier to remember. The categories covered in this text are:
- Overview
- Epidemiologic Concepts of Disease
- Measures of Frequency and Association
- Basic Epidemiologic Methodology
- Observational Studies
- Bias and Error
- Causality
- Surveillance

Each category begins with a short introduction that gives an overview of the principles covered within the category. The series of principles follows in separate modules. Each module contains the statement of the principle and a brief explanation of the principle. One or more examples are given to enhance the understanding of the principle along with definitions of terms. At the end of each module, a brief list of references and closely related principles is given. In addition to the reference lists, there are classic citations. These citations are considered "classic" by the author in that they are some of the most commonly referenced sources in most epidemiologic books.

Mary E. Torrence

FDA, Rockville, Maryland

Contents

Overview

Of this we may be sure, that science, in obeying the law of humanity, will always labor to enlarge the frontiers of life.

Louis Pasteur

There will always be disease in the world, as well as a constant pursuit to understand and conquer its deadly outcome. There will always be medical professionals and scientists driven by their passion for that understanding to have power over disease. Epidemiology is a basic science that can train medical professionals and scientists alike in the skills and analytic reasoning to pursue and understand the distribution, the determinants, and the causes of disease. In that understanding, prevention and control of disease can be implemented. Epidemiology is the study of **Disease Occurrence and Risk Factors of Disease or any health-related event in a Population.** The population may be any group, human or animal. The study of epidemiology incorporates **Critical Reasoning,** research methodology, and statistical analyses to study disease or health-event occurrences in a population and to determine the cause of the disease. These skills may be used in the study of infectious, occupational, environmental, or chronic diseases or even in the study of such fields as psychology. Epidemiology is characterized by its **Interdisciplinary Nature.**

Epidemiology is the basic science of **Population Medicine** and public health and ultimately is used to accomplish the protection of public health. Once the cause of disease and the risk factors for disease are determined, then **Prevention and Control** programs can be implemented. Finally, epidemiologic methods can also be used to measure the success of these prevention programs in reducing disease and can be used in determining health policy directed toward the protection of public health. This overview chapter explains the concepts of epidemiology and what the field is able to accomplish. The rest of the chapters cover the methods of epidemiology.

List of Principles

Disease Occurrence and Risk Factors in Populations
Epidemiology is the study of the occurrence and the risk factors of disease or health-related events in a population and the application of this knowledge to the control of that disease or event.

Critical Reasoning
Epidemiology is a science of creative, critical thinking. Information or data are examined systematically, and conclusions are drawn.

Population Medicine
Epidemiology is the study of disease and its treatment, control, and prevention in a population of individuals, as opposed to clinical medicine, which treats a disease on an individual level. The samples of the populations that are studied must be representative of the population for the results to be generalized to the total population.

Prevention and Control
Part of the discipline of epidemiology is the application of the knowledge gained from the study of a disease to the control or prevention of that disease in a population. Primary prevention is targeted at keeping the disease from occurring. Secondary prevention is targeted at persons in the early stages of disease to keep the disease from progressing. Tertiary prevention is applied at the advanced disease level to prevent disability.

Interdisciplinary Nature
The epidemiologic study of a disease can involve knowledge and methodology from other scientific fields to help determine the cause or risk factors of a disease. Likewise, epidemiologic concepts and methods can be used in other disciplines of scientific study.

Disease Occurrence and Risk Factors in Populations

Epidemiology is the study of the occurrence and the risk factors of disease or health-related events in a population and the application of this knowledge to the control of that disease or event.

Explanation

The definitions of epidemiology are as varied as the terminology used in this field, but the most encompassing one is *"study of the distribution and determinants of health-related states or events in specified populations, and the application of this study to control of health problems."** From this definition all of the important categories and principles of epidemiology develop and will be discussed in this book.

Epidemiology is considered the basic science of public health. Epidemiology incorporates deductive and systematic reasoning, research methodology, and statistical analysis as tools in the description and discovery of the cause of disease. The study of disease begins with creative, yet logical, and systematic reasoning of the current information about the disease of interest and applies this reasoning and epidemiologic skills to define, explain, and solve the mysteries surrounding the cause of disease.

The first step in determining the cause of disease is to describe and measure the distribution of disease in the affected population. This involves defining a case and then describing *who* has the disease and *when* and *where* the population is infected (Chapter 2). The definition of a case is the determination of what characteristics or symptoms define an affected or diseased individual or the population to be studied. Rates are used to measure the frequency of disease in a population, and then adjusted rates or calculated ratios are used to compare the frequencies of different populations to estimate differences and to formulate and test hypotheses about the distribution of disease (Chapter 3).

An important process in determining the cause of disease is to decide what determinants are risk factors for that disease. Determinants are variables that ascertain the nature or outcome. In other words, they are variables that affect the occurrence of a disease or an event. Important clues may come from the study of the natural history or progression of the disease over time and how it is transmitted through the population. Descriptive epidemiologic studies can also provide clues to possible risk factors and help form hypotheses about the cause of a disease. A hypoth-

*Last, J.M. 1988. A Dictionary of Epidemiology. Second edition. Oxford University Press, New York. page 42.

esis is an informed guess. Specific analytic epidemiologic studies are designed to test the proposed hypotheses about the cause of a disease. These studies can also measure the association of the risk factors to disease and the magnitude of that association (Chapters 4 and 5). Finally, certain criteria are applied to help epidemiologists critically examine the evidence and determine if the associated risk factor is actually a *cause* of the disease (Chapter 6). Standard research methods and statistical analysis are helpful tools in developing and testing hypotheses.

The ultimate goal of epidemiology is to explain the occurrences of disease within a population. Most studies, with the exception of perhaps the census, involve studying a "sample" or portion of the population. Thus it is important that the conclusions about a disease and its risk factors in the sample are also true of the general population at risk. The estimates from the sample must be accurate, precise, reliable, and valid to make some conclusions. This involves ensuring against bias and error (Chapter 8).

Epidemiology also includes the application of epidemiologic study to the control of health problems. Control of disease is important in the protection of the public health. Surveillance is an important epidemiologic effort in the prevention and control of disease since it aids in the identification of new or increased occurrences of disease. Rapid and accurate identification is important to initiate control programs in a population. Surveillance can also evaluate the effect of prevention and control programs that have been implemented in a population (Chapter 7).

Example

Examples of epidemiology in action are everyday occurrences. The most commonly used example of an outbreak of disease and the role of epidemiology is a foodborne disease outbreak associated with a church picnic. A large number of individuals attend a church picnic in the summer and 6 to 24 hours later become severely ill with gastrointestinal symptoms that include vomiting, diarrhea, chills, nausea, and a fever. First, investigators must agree on a definition of a case. Which symptoms are considered part of the illness? A case definition could be those individuals that experience vomiting (more than two times in 24 hours), nausea, chills, and diarrhea (more than three bowel movements in 24 hours) 6 or more hours after attending the church picnic. A case definition enables the epidemiologists to measure the frequency of disease in the population. Counts are taken of how many people attended the picnic, how many got sick, and when and what the people ate and drank. For instance, 80 people attended the picnic. Of these, 55 people got sick approximately 6 to 10 hours after the picnic. Of the 55, all of them ate the potato salad, 10 also ate the ham sandwiches, 4 ate hamburgers, and 2 ate the chicken salad. From the information about how many were ill, when they became ill, and what the individuals ate, a

TERMS

Epidemiology	The study of the distribution and the risk factors of disease or health-related events in a population and the application of this knowledge to the control of the disease or event
Distribution	Frequency or occurrence over space and time
Determinants	Factors that determine the outcome or the condition of something
Disease	Absence of health
Public Health	The efforts of society to protect, promote, and restore a population's health

hypothesis can be made about what might be the cause of the disease. Then samples can be taken from the suspected foods and from the ill and non-ill people and tested in the laboratories for evidence to prove the hypothesis. In this case, the potato salad was contaminated with bacteria that caused foodborne disease in the people who consumed it.

Related Principles
Critical reasoning
Interdisciplinary
Population medicine
Prevention and control
Case definition (Epidemiologic concepts of disease)
Person, place, time (Epidemiologic concepts of disease)
Natural history of disease (Epidemiologic concepts of disease)
Modes of transmission (Epidemiologic concepts of disease)
Incidence, prevalence (Measures of frequency and association)
Epidemic, endemic (Measures of frequency and association)
Relative risk (Measures of frequency and association)
Odds ratio (Measures of frequency and association)
Attributable risk (Measures of frequency and association)
Objective and hypothesis (Basic epidemiologic methodology)
Case-control, retrospective studies (Observational studies)
Prospective, cohort studies (Observational studies)
Causation (Causality)

Surveillance versus monitoring (Surveillance)
Active versus passive (Surveillance)
Screening (Surveillance)
Confounding (Bias and error)
Selection bias (Bias and error)
Information bias (Bias and error)
Error (Bias and error)

References

Last, J.M. (ed). 1988. A dictionary of epidemiology. Second Edition. Oxford University Press, New York.

Pleasurable reading for a thorough understanding of epidemiology at work:

1. Cook, Robin. 1982. Fever. G.P. Putnam and Sons. New York. Outbreak. 1987. Berkley Books, New York.
2. Garrett, Laura. 1994. The coming plague. Farrar, Straus, Giroux, New York.
3. Gregg, C.T. 1983. A virus of love and other tales of medical detection. Charles Scribner's Sons, New York.
4. Marr, John, and Cravens, Gwyneth. 1977. Black death. Ballentine, New York.
5. Percy, Walker. 1987. The thanatos syndrome. Farrar, Straus, Giroux, New York.
6. Roueche, Berton. 1980, 1982. Medical detectives I and II. Washington Square Press, Pocket Books, a division of Simon and Schuster, New York.
7. Roueche, Berton. 1971. The orange man. Little, Brown, and Company. Boston, Massachusetts.
8. Roueche, Berton. 1968. Eleven blue men. Berkeley Medalion Books, New York.
9. Roueche, Berton. 1967. Annals of epidemiology. Little, Brown, and Company. Boston, Massachusetts.

Critical Reasoning

Epidemiology is a science of creative, critical thinking. Information or data are examined systematically, and conclusions are drawn.

Explanation

One of the most difficult concepts to comprehend when first studying epidemiology is that it involves a way of thinking rather than, like many of the other medical fields, a great deal of memorization. Part of the study of epidemiology is the process of training the mind to think critically. Although many think epidemiology involves only statistics and formulas, it is really a systematic way of reasoning to solve a problem, generally the cause of disease. This critical reasoning involves beginning with a general, broad problem, collecting information about the problem, and then solving the problem by studying the specific information collected.

Epidemiologists are faced with new diseases that emerge, sudden large increases of a disease in a population, or diseases that persist in high numbers over many years despite knowledge about their cause and their risk factors. Epidemiologists search for answers. Critical and systematic thinking helps epidemiologists design methods to study the problems, collect more information, and make accurate conclusions.

This type of reasoning is important in epidemiologic studies but is also valuable to medical professionals and researchers in analyzing journal articles and scientific reports. During medical training, the emphasis is on clinical treatment, not on research methods and analysis. How does a clinician decide to use a new treatment or drug? Is it by reading journal articles, listening to drug salespersons, or listening to a seminar given at a conference? How does that clinician know that the information is correct and that the new treatment is safe and effective? Most clinicians, whether they realize it or not, make some kind of informed, logical choice. Deductive and critical reasoning can help make a scientific and knowledgeable decision.

When reading medical articles, questions should be asked:

What is the objective or purpose of the study?

Is the study design appropriate to answer the objective?

What is being measured? Is it defined?

Is the sample appropriate and large enough to make conclusions about the affected population?

What sources of bias or error can occur?

How is the information collected?

Is the information standardized if it is collected by more than one researcher or facility?

How are the data analyzed? Are the statistics appropriate for the type of data collected?

Are the findings consistent?

Do the tables and graphs make sense?

Do the data justify the conclusions?

Analysis of the focused areas of these questions can give readers of journal articles important information to make informed, scientific decisions about the quality of the study. The quality of the study determines the credibility of the conclusions.

Example

In the spring of 1993 the U.S. Center for Disease Control and Prevention (CDC) reported 24 cases of acute respiratory illness that resulted in death in several people in Arizona, Colorado, New Mexico, and Utah. The ages of those affected ranged from young to old. Fatalities were more than 50%. The cases seemed to be localized in this one specific geographic area. This new disease elicited rapid action by various health agencies to determine the cause of the disease. What would you do?

Careful and systematic reasoning started an investigation into the characteristics of the people affected and possible exposures. The ages of those affected ranged from 12 to 69 years old, with males and females affected. Various ethnic groups were affected, with the American Indian being disproportionately affected. Although the cases were originally located in the 4 states, other cases occurred in 14 other states including California, Oregon, and the northern Midwest. Most of the affected individuals lived in rural areas.

A search was conducted for the organism. It was finally identified from affected tissues through various laboratory tests. It was a new strain of the Hantavirus. Once the organism was discovered, investigations were needed to determine the source of the organism. Testing was done of the environment and any small animals. The Hantavirus was isolated from deer mouse tissues in November 1993. This small mammal resides in many parts of the United States. People at risk for Hantavirus pulmonary syndrome are those that might come in close contact with the excreta of the mouse. The isolation of the virus has enabled diagnostic testing to be developed to diagnose future cases. Hantavirus has emerged as a new important disease in the United States.

TERMS

Deductive Reasoning	Inference, a conclusion is made about a general problem from logical reasoning about the specifics

Related Principles

Disease occurrence and risk factors in populations
Objective and hypothesis (Basic epidemiologic methodology)

References

Blalock, H.M. 1964. Causal inferences in nonexperimental research. Norton, New York.

Buck, M. 1975. Popper's philosophy for epidemiology. Int. J. Epidemiol. 4: 159-168.

Bunge, M. 1979. Causality and modern science. Third edition. Dover, New York. Chapter 1.

Conant, J.B. 1951. Science and common sense. Yale University Press, New Haven, Connecticut. Chapter 3.

Popper, K.R. 1968. The logic of scientific discovery. Harper and Row, New York.

Susser, M. 1973. Causal thinking in the health sciences. Oxford University Press, New York.

Walker, A.M. 1991. Observation and inference: an introduction to the methods of epidemiology. Epidemiology Resources Inc, Chestnut Hill, Massachusetts.

Population Medicine

Epidemiology is the study of disease and its treatment, control, and prevention in a population of individuals, as opposed to clinical medicine, which treats a disease on an individual level. The samples of the populations that are studied must be representative of the population for the results to be generalized to the total population.

Explanation

Practitioners of clinical medicine study disease and recommend treatment for individual patients. In contrast, epidemiology is the study of disease and treatment in a group of individuals or population. Each medical discipline offers important information to the other in the study of disease. Information about a disease or treatment collected at the population level can also be used on a diseased individual. Likewise, clinical history and laboratory tests of diseased individuals offer important clues in determining risk factors for a disease in the general population.

The study of populations offers some challenges. The first step is to define the population. The defined population may be a group with a specific characteristic or a group exposed to a specific event. For example, specific group characteristics that are studied include biological characteristics, such as race or families or twin; special religious or cultural characteristics; or demographic characteristics, such as age or gender. Specific events that occur in a group could include geographic location, occupation, or natural disasters. The information that is collected is not about individuals but is a summary of all individuals in the population and their patterns and characteristics. Conclusions based on the population information cannot be automatically applied to an individual.

It is nearly impossible in a laboratory situation or even in epidemiologic studies to observe the entire population. It is more common to study a sample of the population. Studying a proportion of the population of interest is not useful unless the data collected are applicable at the population level; therefore the sample must be representative of the potentially affected total population. The sampled proportion of the population should be similar in the characteristics of interest, demographics, and any other attribute that might have an influence on the study. The sampled proportion must also have the same opportunity to become diseased or to be exposed to the event of interest as the general population. If the sampled population is representative of the general population, then the data obtained from the study may be *carefully* applied or generalized to the total population.

Examples

1. Seventh-Day Adventists are a particular religious population that believe in abstinence from the use of tobacco and alcohol. They are often studied and compared to smokers and drinkers to determine the effects of such risk factors like smoking and alcohol on disease. 2. There is a need to learn the effects of exposures to certain particulates or fumes in the air on the occurrence of asthma. A study is designed to look at the frequency of asthma in certain occupational groups, such as workers in chemical, rubber, metal industry, and stone, glass, and concrete product plants.

TERMS

Demographics	The statistical study of a population in regards to the distribution, number, vital statistics, and characteristics such as age, gender, race, occupation, and socioeconomic status
Generalization	The act of taking specific information and applying it on a more general basis
Inference	Conclusions made about a population based on results from a sample or subgroup
Population	Total number of people in a specific area or having a similar characteristic
Representative	A typical sample of a group or characteristic that can stand for another

Related Principles

Critical reasoning
Disease occurrence and risk factors in populations
Herd immunity (Epidemiologic concepts of disease)
Cross-sectional, survey studies (Observational studies)
Attributable risk (Measures of frequency and association)
Natural, ecologic studies (Observational studies)

References

Redfern, P. 1989. Population registers: some administrative and statistical pros and cons. J. Royal Statistical Society, Series A. 152:1-41.

Prevention and Control

Part of the discipline of epidemiology is the application of the knowledge gained from the study of a disease to the control or prevention of that disease in a population. Primary prevention is targeted at keeping the disease from occurring. Secondary prevention is targeted at persons in the early stages of disease to keep the disease from progressing. Tertiary prevention is applied at the advanced disease level to prevent disability.

Explanation

Epidemiology not only involves the study of disease in populations but also the application of prevention or control programs in that population. Although epidemiologists strive to determine the cause and associated risk factors of a disease, the ultimate conquest of disease is achieved through prevention or at least control of the disease in a population. Prevention and control of the disease in the population also lead to prevention and control on an individual patient level. Preventive measures keep a disease from occurring. Control of a disease involves the management of the disease in an individual so that it does not progress or the prevention of the spread of the disease in a population. An expanded definition of prevention includes the control of disease.

How does epidemiology contribute to the prevention of disease? Epidemiology provides a method for describing and defining the natural history of disease and for determining risk factors for disease. Once risk factors have been determined, intervention trials can be used to determine what changes in the risk factor affect the incidence of a disease. Intervention trials are aimed at altering one or more of the risk factors for a disease in a limited sample of the population. Epidemiologic inquiry is important in determining the modes of transmission of disease. This is essential knowledge for the prevention of disease in a population.

Several levels of prevention are aimed at different stages of disease. The primary level involves the prevention of the disease from occurring by either altering the exposure or the susceptibility of the individual. Primary prevention is aimed at the time of exposure or infection. The secondary prevention level involves early detection of disease and treatment. Secondary prevention is aimed at the very early stages of a disease. The tertiary prevention level involves the prevention of disability from disease and rehabilitation. Tertiary prevention can only be used in stages of advanced disease.

Primary prevention is the ideal goal but is not often achieved. It includes two methods of prevention, general promotion measures and specific protective measures. General health promotion includes low-fat diets and exercise to prevent heart disease. It includes efforts for a safe workplace and home to protect against occupational hazards and accidents. Health education is needed to implement other protective measures such as good nutrition, adequate shelter, immunization, sanitation, and safe water. Immunization and good sanitation practices are common primary preventive measures against infectious diseases especially in developed countries. Primary prevention is more difficult in other diseases, such as heart disease, stroke, human immunodeficiency virus, sexually-transmitted diseases, and injuries, because prevention not only depends on science and new technology but also on behavior modification. Behavior changes in a population are difficult to achieve unless the individuals are motivated. No one has determined how to prevent deaths resulting from guns or automobile accidents.

Secondary prevention is the diagnosis or detection of early disease and the prevention of disease progression. Efforts include curing the disease, slowing the progression with treatment, preventing complications and disabilities, and reversing communicability among the population. To prevent disease progression, the disease must be detected in the early stages. Screening programs are used to detect disease early in an individual. The early detection of infected individuals allows treatment of those individuals and ultimately prevents the spread of disease, if it is communicable, from those individuals to others in the population. Secondary prevention efforts are more common than primary efforts because many diseases cannot be prevented, such as diabetes. Diabetes can be treated to prevent the progression of the disease.

Tertiary prevention is the prevention of disability from advanced disease or the rehabilitation of an individual with a chronic disease. These efforts involve restoring an affected individual to maximum potential and usefulness. These efforts involve not only medical but also psychologic and vocational efforts. Stroke is one disease that would require tertiary prevention.

Once prevention or control measures have been implemented, epidemiology can also help evaluate the impact of those measures. Epidemiology can provide the method for study of the effect of prevention and control programs on the occurrence of a disease in a population. Studies can evaluate the occurrence and distribution of a disease in a population before and after a prevention program. A comparison of these numbers can show a positive or negative effect of the program on a disease. This information can help evaluate the effectiveness and the benefit of the program.

TERMS

Control	To reduce the incidence or prevalence of disease; have influence over disease
Intervention	To interfere with or hinder the progression of disease
Prevention	The promotion, preservation, and restoration of health; to keep disease from occurring
Primary Prevention	The prevention of disease from occurring
Secondary Prevention	The prevention of progression of early-staged disease
Tertiary Prevention	Prevention of disability from advanced disease and the rehabilitation of the individual to functional capacity

Examples
1. Primary prevention level
   a. Water fluoridation to prevent dental caries.
   b. Immunization of children against certain infectious diseases, such as diphtheria, whooping cough, and measles.
   c. Vaccination of domestic animals against rabies to prevent infection and further spread of rabies to humans.

2. Secondary prevention level
   a. Mammographic screening for early signs of breast cancer.
   b. Cholesterol testing for high levels to prevent heart disease.
   c. Screening for high blood pressure to prevent stroke.
3. Tertiary prevention level
   a. Rehabilitation of stroke and head-injury cases.
   b. Rehabilitation of polio victims.
   c. Rehabilitation of paralyzed individuals.

Related Principles

Screening (Surveillance)
Natural history of disease (Epidemiologic concepts of disease)
Modes of transmission (Epidemiologic concepts of disease)
Herd immunity (Epidemiologic concepts of disease)
Attributable risk (Measures of frequency and association)

References

Caplan, G., Grunebaum, H. 1967. Perspectives on primary prevention: a review. Arch. Gen. Psychiat. 17:331-346.
Wall, S. 1995. Epidemiology for prevention. Int. J. Epidemiol. 24:655-664.
Walter, S.D. 1980. Prevention for multifactorial disease. Am. J. Epidemiol. 112:409-416.
Wegman, D.H. 1992. The potential impact of epidemiology on the prevention of occupational disease. Am. J. Public Health 8:944-954.

Interdisciplinary Science

The epidemiologic study of a disease can involve knowledge and methodology from other scientific fields to help determine the cause or risk factors of a disease. Likewise, epidemiologic concepts and methods can be used in other disciplines of scientific study.

Explanation

The art of epidemiology involves and incorporates various disciplines of study to solve the puzzle of the cause or the risk factors of a disease or an event. New technologies have added to the success of epidemiologic endeavors. For example, molecular techniques have opened limitless possibilities for epidemiologic studies. Technologies, such as nucleic acid-based methods, help identify new pathogens.

The development of monoclonal antibodies has allowed epidemiologists to differentiate among rabies viruses in different geographic regions. Each geographic region usually has one specific animal species that is responsible for the maintenance of the disease in the population. Each animal reservoir has a specific strain of the virus (ecotype) that shows a distinct monoclonal antibody pattern. The immunofluorescent reaction of a monoclonal antibody panel results in a characteristic pattern for each rabies virus ecotype. The pattern tells epidemiologists the possible source of the rabies infection. This technology enabled epidemiologists to determine that the origin of the raccoon rabies epidemic in the mid-Atlantic region was a result of translocated rabid raccoons from the rabies that was endemic in Florida. This new technology is useful in human rabies cases when there is no recollection of exposure to a rabid animal.

Clinical medicine and pathology are often important for describing a disease and determining possible risk factors. Veterinarians and food scientists may be involved in the study of infectious or foodborne diseases. Counselors and psychologists may be involved in determining the risk factors for diseases involving behavior such as depression and violence. Nutritionists use their expertise to determine if specific nutrients are involved in the development or treatment of a particular disease. Epidemiologic methods enable the study of a wide range of diseases and the involvement with others in various disciplines. This is exciting to epidemiologists who seem to have an incredible curiosity and a desire to pursue and answer many questions. In addition, the basic skills of epidemiology expand with new technologies. Early in the history of epidemiology, epidemiologists performed what has been referred to as "shoeleather epidemiology." This term came from the fact that epidemiologists often walked from one area to another tracking new cases of disease and possible sources of infection. This is still done, but as the technology and computer age have exploded, epidemiologists find themselves using computerized patient records to track new cases or to communicate with other epidemiologists.

The analytic and research methodology and the reasoning learned in epidemiology can be applied to almost any field of study involving health or disease. Epidemiologic studies are used in health psychology to study diseases that are caused or can be reduced by health behaviors. Observational studies are also used to explore the risk factors for depression and violence. New subspecialties of epidemiology continue to appear in the literature. For example, molecular epidemiology helps in the study of the incidence of antibiotic resistance and its role in disease in humans and foodborne diseases. Pharmacoepidemiology studies how drugs and drug-interactions might cause disease in people.

Examples

1. CDC has established a new center to study the epidemiology of violent behavior in the United States. This will involve surveillance of certain types of violence, such as domestic violence and handgun injuries, and epidemiologic studies to explore the risk factors for violence.

2. The multistate outbreak of *E. coli 0157:H7* infections from hamburgers in the western United States caused numerous fatalities. To determine the cause and source of this foodborne disease many different disciplines were involved in a joint effort to solve the problem. Epidemiologists and public health officials collected information on those infected after clinicians alerted the health departments. Laboratory personnel were involved in testing infected individuals, samples from those individuals, and suspected foods for the presence of an organism. Veterinarians were involved in determining the risk factors for infection during animal processing and the risk factors for prevention of further contamination of food. Food hygienists were essential for determining the proper methods for food processing in preventing the outbreaks.

Related Principles

Disease occurrence and risk factors in populations

References

Fletcher, R.H., Fletcher, S.W., and Wagner, E.H. 1982. Clinical epidemiology-the essentials. Williams & Wilkins, Baltimore, Maryland.

Kaplan, R.M., and Criqui, M.J. (eds.). 1985. Behavioral epidemiology and disease prevention. Plenum Publishers, New York.

Kewitz, H. 1987. Epidemiological concepts in clinical pharmacology. Springer-Verlag, New York.

Martin, S.W., Meek, A.H., and Willeberg, P. 1987. Veterinary epidemiology: principles and methods. Iowa State University Press, Ames, Iowa.

Monson, R.R. 1990. Occupational epidemiology. Second edition. CRC Press, New York.

Morris, J.N. 1975. Uses of epidemiology. Third edition. E.S. Livingstone, London, England.

Morton, N.E., and Chung, C.S., (eds.). 1978. Genetic epidemiology. Oxford University Press, New York.

Omenn, G.S. 1993. The role of environmental epidemiology in public policy. Ann. Epidemiol. 3:318-322.

Schoenberg, B.S. (ed.). 1978. Neurological epidemiology: principles and clinical applications. Raven Press, New York.

Smith, R.D. 1991. Veterinary clinical epidemiology: a problem-oriented approach. Buttersworth-Heinermainn, Stoneham, Massachusetts.

Stephenson, J. 1996. Disease detectives are turning to molecular techniques to uncover emerging microbes. JAMA 275(3):176.

Valanis, B. 1986. Epidemiology in nursing and health care. Appleton & Lange, New York.

TERMS

Interdisciplinary	Several disciplines interact with each other. Principles and methods from one discipline can be used in the study of another discipline
Endemic	A constant or steady level of disease in a certain geographic area or population

Overview: Study Questions

1. Select a scientific article in a recent journal. Critically evaluate the objective, design, analysis, and conclusions of the study. What is your conclusion about the results?
2. Explain the major components of the basic science of epidemiology and describe three different fields in which epidemiology can be used.
3. When is it more appropriate to draw conclusions from a sample of a population than from the entire population at risk?
4. Define one or two populations to be used for the study of two different diseases or exposures of interest. Justify your selection of the populations.
5. Why is it important for a sample of the population to be representative of the general population?
6. Name the three different levels of prevention and give examples of diseases, other than those mentioned in the text, that could be affected by each level of prevention.
7. What prevention level is addressed by screening programs and how?
8. Name five different fields of study in which epidemiologic methods and reasoning would be useful in the study of a problem.
9. Describe three different fields, other than those mentioned in the text, that would contribute to the epidemiologic study of disease.
10. Describe two new technologies or advances, other than those mentioned in the text, that could contribute to epidemiology in the future.

CHAPTER 2

Epidemiologic Concepts of Disease

The medical concepts relevant to disease and health-related events are already familiar to those in the biomedical sciences. However, there are specific epidemiologic concepts essential to the understanding and study of disease. These concepts are useful in the understanding of any disease or any event such as an automobile accident, that might be health-related. Disease is considered the lack of health. In any disease investigation, whether it is to determine if there is an outbreak, whether it is to estimate the frequency and severity of the illness, or whether it is to determine the causes of disease, the starting point is to define what entity is being counted. The **Case Definition** of the entity or case is an exposure, disease, or health-related event. Once cases have been defined, then simple descriptions of the distributions of characteristics such as **Person, Place, and Time,** can provide a better understanding of the epidemiology of the disease and help formulate hypotheses about the cause of disease. Both case definition and the distribution of person, place, and time are important in understanding the disease and for further study. If the disease is new, an understanding of the **Natural History of Disease** and how the disease is transmitted within a population can help in the determination of the etiology of the disease. Knowledge of how the disease progresses and is transmitted is useful in designing intervention and control programs. If the disease is infectious, its perpetuation in the population depends on the **Modes of Transmission** of the disease from infected individuals to susceptible individuals. If there are very few susceptible individuals among a largely immune population, then the likelihood of these individuals becoming infected would be small. This phenomenon, or **Herd Immunity,** is important in understanding the course of a disease in the population and has been applied for the control or prevention of some infectious diseases. Although many of these concepts in this chapter are specific or more relevant to infectious diseases that are on the rise, these principles can also be applied to noninfectious diseases, such as environmental, occupational, and chronic diseases.

List of Principles

Case Definition   A clear, concise definition of what is considered a case is essential for knowing what to measure. Measurement of the frequency and distribution of the disease in a population is necessary to the understanding and study of the causes of disease. The concise definition allows a relatively standardized comparison of cases among different groups so that each group is measuring the same entity.

Person, Place, and Time   Descriptive epidemiology is used to describe the distribution of the event of interest in terms of the person, place, and time affected in a population. The description of disease in terms of the people affected, the place and time in which the disease occurs, are important in determining the possible etiology of the disease and risk factors affecting the disease. These three variables can also be important risk factors for disease.

Natural History of Disease   The natural history of disease is the course of a disease without intervention from the time of exposure to the resolution of the disease in an individual or population. Understanding the stages of the natural history of disease is vital in applying epidemiologic principles to detect and diagnose disease, to determine the etiology of disease, and to prevent or control transmission of the disease.

Modes of Transmission   Determining the mode of transmission of disease is critical to understanding the epidemiology of the disease, its survival in the population, and methods of control. The distribution of person, place, and time of the disease in the population can help formulate hypotheses about the mode of transmission of disease of an unknown etiology.

Herd Immunity   Herd immunity describes the ability to protect susceptible individuals in a group from disease by the presence of a high proportion of immune individuals in the same population. Whether the susceptible individuals are infected depends on how many immune individuals are in the population and how likely the susceptibles are to come into contact with an infected individual. The concept of herd immunity is used to control and prevent disease in populations.

Case Definition

A clear, concise definition of what is considered a case is essential for knowing what to measure. Measurement of the frequency and distribution of the disease in a population is necessary to the understanding and study of the causes of disease. The concise definition allows a relatively standardized comparison of cases among different groups so that each group is measuring the same entity.

Explanation

By medical definition, a case is an individual or animal that is diseased. A single case, however, in epidemiologic terms, can be an exposure, a disease, or a health-related event. A definition for what is considered a case is important in epidemiologic study. For example, 40 out of 50 people at a catered barbecue become ill with gastrointestinal symptoms 12 hours after the event. A case would be an individual who is ill. In a different situation, there is an infected individual with tuberculosis who is treated at a local hospital without special precautions. The important issue would be to determine exposures and follow these individuals in time to see if they become infected. A case would be an individual exposed to the infected individual. A case definition is clear, concise criteria for inclusion and measurement as a case. The criteria can be highly restrictive or very broad depending on how many and what types of cases need to be measured. For example, if every possible case of influenza needs to be measured, then the criteria would be broad and would include all flulike symptoms, in addition to cases with symptoms of respiratory disease and gastrointestinal disease. If health officials only want to determine more definite influenza cases, then the criteria would be more restrictive and would only include those individuals with flulike symptoms. To count cases, there must be an ability to detect and diagnose disease. Because detection and diagnosis can be difficult in latent or subclinical disease, diagnostic criteria may be included in the criteria for a case definition; these include clinical symptoms and laboratory values.

Once a case definition is established, then you can determine cases and noncases of disease; this will allow you to determine if there is a true outbreak of disease or the occurrence of a new disease.

A standardized case definition gives you a valid measurement from various sources of the distribution of cases in a population and allows comparisons of these measures among groups. Comparing two groups or measurements that are not alike will give you wrong information. A standardized case definition helps to establish that everyone refers to a certain disease in the same way. A patient may be diagnosed with Lyme disease in one area of the United States and not the other. Standardization is so important that in 1948 the World Health Organization (WHO) developed the International Classification of Diseases (ICD) codes so that the coding of diseases in medical charts and on death certificates by various medical professionals would be standardized. If the criteria are not clear, it is possible the cases may be misclassified as noncases or noncases may be misclassified as cases. These incorrect numbers can affect conclusions about the distribution of the disease in the population.

Changes in case definition are important to note when looking at trends in disease over time. Changes in the criteria may cause a temporary increase or decrease in numbers reported but are not necessarily a true increase in the disease.

Example

The United States Centers for Disease Control and Prevention (CDC) maintains a surveillance of certain reportable diseases, and each state is responsible for reporting these diseases. Therefore CDC has established a standard case definition for each disease so that all states are consistent in reporting.

In 1983 CDC established a case definition for a previously unknown disease, acquired immune deficiency syndrome (AIDS). The case definition was expanded in 1987 and in 1993 to reflect the increasing knowledge. The 1993 expanded definition includes all persons infected with the human immunodeficiency virus (HIV) having less than 200 CD4 + T-lymphocytes/uL or a CD4 + T-lymphocyte percentage of total lymphocytes of less than 14 and three more clinical conditions, pulmonary tuberculosis, recurrent pneumonia, and invasive cervical cancer. CDC's objective for expanding the AIDS case definition was to detect HIV-infected individuals earlier that were otherwise asymptomatic, to more accurately capture HIV morbidity and immunosuppression. This would give a better picture of the HIV epidemic because current drugs have delayed symptoms of the disease and therefore reflect a lower number of reported cases. Also, women who were infected with HIV had a different clinical picture than the more typical HIV-infected men.

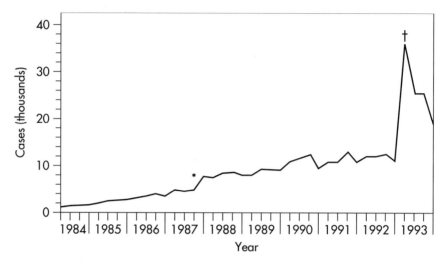

Fig. 2-1   AIDS cases, by quarter year of report, in the United States, 1984 to 1993.
* In October 1987 the case definition and diagnostic criteria were revised.
+ In 1993 the case definition was revised again. (From CDC. 1994. Update: Trends in AIDS diagnosis and reporting under the expanded surveillance definition for adolescents and adults—United States, 1993. MMWR 43(32):826-828.)

The immediate effect of this change in definition was to cause an increase in the number of reported cases because of the inclusion of the existing cases of AIDS that were not previously diagnosed or reported. This is clearly demonstrated in Fig. 2-1. Over time the trend will level off because both new and existing cases will be reported and not just new cases under the definition.

TERMS

Case

A person within a population that according to the criteria established is identified as having a particular disease, exposure, or event. The epidemiologic definition of a case is not necessarily the clinical definition.

Related Principles
Numerator, denominator (Measures of frequency and association)
Incidence, prevalence (Measures of frequency and association)
Selection bias (Bias and error)
Case-control, retrospective studies (Observational studies)

References

CDC. 1987. Revision of the CDC surveillance case definition for acquired immunodeficiency syndrome. MMWR 36: Number 1S.

CDC. 1992. 1993 revised classification system for HIV infection and expanded surveillance case definition for AIDS among adolescents and adults. MMWR 41:RR-17.

CDC, Update. 1994. Impact of the expanded AIDS surveillance case definition for adolescents and adults on case reporting: U.S., 1993. MMWR 43:160-161, 167-170.

Lilienfield, A.M., and Lilienfield, D.E. 1980. Foundations of epidemiology. Second edition. Oxford University Press, New York. Revised by Lilienfield, D.E., and Stolley, P.D. (eds.) 1994. Foundations of epidemiology. Third edition. Oxford University Press, New York.

Mausner, J.S., and Kramer, S. 1985. Mausner and Bahn, Epidemiology: an introductory text. WB Saunders Co. Philadelphia, Pennsylvania.

Schlesselman, J.J. 1982. Case control studies: design, conduct, analysis. Monographs in epidemiology and biostatistics, Vol. 2. Oxford University Press, New York.

Person, Place, and Time

Descriptive epidemiology is used to describe the distribution of the event of interest in terms of the person, place, and time affected in a population. The description of disease in terms of the people affected, the place and time in which the disease occurs, are important in determining the possible etiology of the disease and risk factors affecting the disease. These three variables can also be important risk factors for disease.

Explanation

Person is studied by the distribution patterns of age, gender, race, socioeconomic status, and occupation (e.g., occupational epidemiology) in an affected population. The study of these factors, or demography, and their influence on behavior, healthcare, and even detection of disease, are too complex for this text; however, all of these factors also influence differences in disease occurrence in populations and must be considered in the design and analysis of epidemiologic studies. Age is the most important factor; for almost any disease, age affects the mortality and morbidity rates. The very young and old are more susceptible because of an underdeveloped or compromised immune system. When calculating the mortality rates according to age, the graph is a characteristic J-shaped curve; that is, the very young and the very old have the highest incidence. The severity of disease or morbidity rates may also have a similar J-shaped curve since the young and the old are most likely

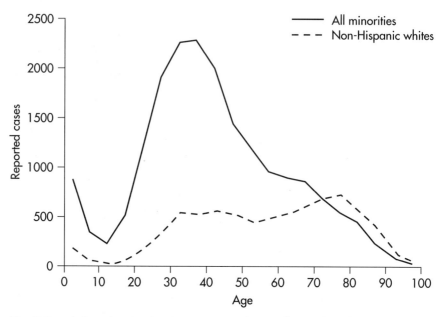

Fig. 2-2   J-shaped curve that is common with mortality and morbidity rates. (Frequency distribution of tuberculosis cases, 1992.) (From CDC. 1993. Summary of notifiable diseases—United States, 1992. MMWR 41(55):1-73.)

to be severely affected by disease. Infectious diseases often have a J-shaped curve.

In Fig. 2-2 a graph of tuberculosis cases shows a J-shaped curve for ages 1 to 40. Those individuals under age 10 and over age 30 are more susceptible to tuberculosis. Tuberculosis is not a common disease in older individuals; therefore the number of cases is not high. On the other hand, influenza is a common disease in the elderly and would show an elevated number of cases and a J-shaped curve.

Gender is also important in mortality and morbidity studies. Males often have higher rates of mortality although females have higher reported rates of morbidity (Fig. 2-3).

Ethnicity is important in that some ethnic groups have a higher prevalence or susceptibility to disease. For example, African Americans have a higher incidence of hypertension and sickle cell anemia than other ethnic groups. These ethnic differences can be studied to explore possible risk factors for disease. Variables related to person are important to consider when comparing rates among different populations. If the populations differ greatly with respect to age or gender, then the populations must be adjusted statistically for comparisons to be made.

Place is most often described by the geographic pattern of the disease

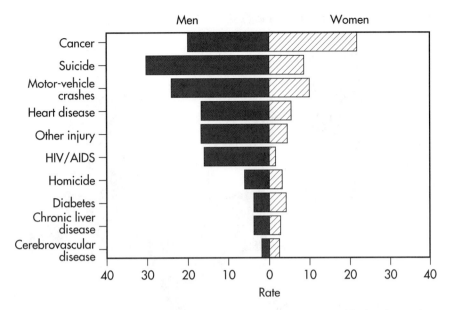

Fig. 2-3 Death rates (per 100,000 persons ages 25 to 44 years old of each sex) for the 10 leading causes of death, by sex—Utah, 1988 to 1992. (From CDC. 1994. Leading causes of death, by age and sex—Utah, 1988-1992. MMWR 43(37):685-687.)

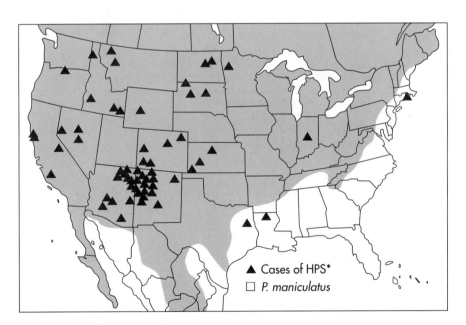

Fig. 2-4 Geographic distribution of the white-footed mouse *(Peromyscus manic-ulatus)* and the number of recognized cases of Hantavirus pulmonary syndrome as of March 23, 1994. (From CDC. 1994. Addressing emerging infectious disease threats: a prevention strategy for the United States Executive Summary. MMWR 43(RR-5):8.)

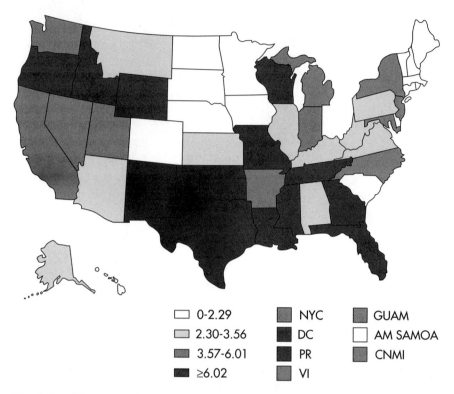

Fig. 2-5   The reported cases (per 100,000) of Hepatitis B in the United States and territories, 1993. (From CDC. 1994. Summary of notifiable diseases—United States, 1993. MMWR 42(53):34.)

or the spatial distribution of the event (Fig. 2-4). Place may be linked to a certain exposure or even a certain physical or biologic attribute of the environment that helps to determine the etiology or risk factors for disease. The distribution may be clustered, localized, or widespread and is depicted by a variety of types of graphs or maps (Fig. 2-5). The type of distribution may give a clue to the etiology of the disease; for example, a localized sickness may be a result of exposure to a chemical. More complex information that is sometimes considered with place is the climate and topographic features.

Time of disease occurrence can be measured in short- or long-term trends. Shorter periods of occurrence such as hours or days are important to analyze especially in occupational diseases where exposure to a risk factor is short. Seasonal patterns of disease are important in determining the transmission of the disease and possible times for intervention or control. Longer or secular trends, usually a year or more, are important in looking at fluctuations in case numbers and in studying dis-

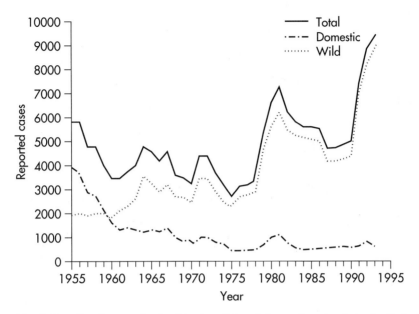

Fig. 2-6   Secular trends of rabies in wild and domestic animals in the United States and Puerto Rico, 1955 to 1993. (From CDC. 1994. Summary of notifiable diseases—United States, 1993. MMWR 42(53):46.)

eases that take a long time before symptoms appear. Changes in secular trends of diseases can be used to measure how well a control program for a particular disease does in reducing the incidence by comparing the rates of disease before and after the intervention. Time is often displayed on graphs of number of cases/events per unit time. It is important to realize that changes in secular trends may reflect other influences other than the true change of disease incidence in mortality or morbidity. Changes in secular trends may be caused by better diagnostic and detection technology or new treatments that either cure the disease or prolong survival (Fig. 2-6). For example, a new diagnostic test would cause an increase in morbidity rates as compared to the time period before the new test. A new treatment that cures a disease would cause a decrease in mortality rates compared to the time period before the new treatment.

Related Principles

Standardization (Measures of frequency and association)
Modes of transmission
Incidence, prevalence (Measures of frequency and association)
Numerator, denominator (Measures of frequency and association)

TERMS

Cluster	A closely grouped series of events or cases in relation to time or place or both
Demographics	The study of the population in regards to the age, size, gender, ethnicity, and other factors of that population
Descriptive Epidemiology	The study or description of the distribution of variables in a population
Morbidity	The number of individuals sick in a population (morbidity number); diseased
Mortality	The number of individuals dead in a population (mortality number); death
Secular	Changes over a long period of time, most often years or even decades
Spatial	Related to occupying space
Spot Map	A map that shows the geographic location of people with a certain characteristic, for example, cases of a disease. It is often used in the investigation of an outbreak

References

Elliott P., Cuzick J., English D., and Stern R. (eds). 1992. Geographical and environmental epidemiology: methods for small-area studies. Oxford University Press, New York. Published on behalf of the World Health Organization Regional Office for Europe.

Lilienfield, A.M., and Lilienfield, D.E. 1980. Foundations of epidemiology. Second edition. Oxford University Press, New York. Revised by Lilienfield, D.E., and Stolley, P.D. (eds.) 1994. Foundations of epidemiology. Third edition. Oxford University Press, New York.

Mausner, J.S., and Kramer, S. 1985. Mausner and Bahn, Epidemiology: an introductory text. WB Saunders Co. Philadelphia, Pennsylvania.

Yorke, J.A., Nathanson, N., Pianigiani G., and Martin, J. 1979. Seasonality and the requirement for perpetuation and eradication of viruses in populations. Am J. of Epidemiol. 109(2):103-123.

Natural History of Disease

The natural history of disease is the course of a disease without intervention from the time of exposure to the resolution of the disease in an individual or population. Understanding the stages of the natural history of disease is vital in applying epidemiologic principles to detect and diagnose disease, to determine the etiology of disease, and to prevent or control transmission of the disease.

Explanation

The natural course of disease includes the following stages: the time from exposure to the onset of disease or incubation period; the time from the onset of disease to the occurrence of clinical symptoms or the subclinical stage; the time from clinical symptoms to diagnosis or the clinical phase; and the time from diagnosis to an outcome such as chronic disease, recovery, or death.

For epidemiologists, the stage of subclinical disease can be a major obstacle in determining the epidemiology of a disease of unknown etiology if there is not a method of detection of a disease or if detection can only be achieved through cumbersome, expensive, screening. At the time of subclinical disease, the individual is infected, yet shows no symptoms. Without detection, estimates of the frequency and distribution of the disease in the population are low and important information about diseased individuals is lost. Subclinical disease is important in the perpetuation of disease in a population because infected individuals can transmit disease to others undetected unless there is a method of detecting subclinical disease.

Latent infections are not as important in transmission because individuals do not normally shed the agent but latent infections are equally difficult to detect. Detection in early stages is almost impossible in slow viruses. For example, kuru or scrapie are slow viruses; therefore determining the epidemiology of these diseases is difficult. Latent infections also make it difficult to measure cases of disease.

The generation period is the time from infection to the period of maximal communicability and is an important consideration in the transmission of disease. Although some consider the generation period to be the same as the incubation period, the generation period can be different. For example, mumps can be transmitted up to 48 hours past the clinical symptoms of swollen salivary glands.

The period of time that it takes to pass from the point of exposure to the onset of clinical illness is often referred to as the incubation period. This period allows the pathogen to multiply inside the host to have

Cases

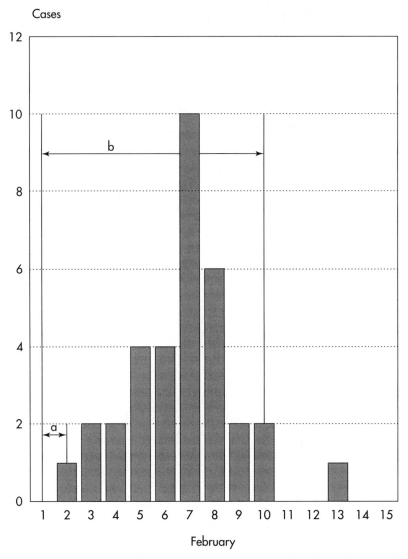

Fig. 2-7   Minimum and maximum incubation periods in hypothetical outbreak in February. *a*, Probable minimum incubation period. *b*, Probable maximum incubation period.

enough numbers to produce clinical illness. Knowing the incubation period can help in estimation of the time of exposure or even the first (index) case, if the onset of disease is known (Fig. 2-7). Because most infectious organisms have characteristic incubation periods, calculating the incubation period may give a clue to the etiology of the disease.

Example

Rabies is an example of a virus that has mastered the art of survival in the wild animal population largely because of its natural history. Incubation periods are varied and prolonged. Subclinical disease is undetectable because the virus travels from the bite wound to the central nervous system via the peripheral nervous system; therefore no virus or antibodies can be detected in the bloodstream. By the time the virus reaches the brain and then travels along the peripheral nervous system to other parts of the body, such as the salivary glands, the host becomes aggressive and irritable, creating a perfect behavior for attacking another animal or human. At this point, the virus is in the salivary glands and can be transmitted to another animal. At the time of appearance of clinical signs, the disease has no treatment and is usually fatal.

TERMS

Generation Period	Time from the receipt of infection to the time of maximal infectivity
Incubation Period	Time from entrance of an infectious agent to the first signs of disease
Induction Period	Term used instead of incubation period in chronic disease epidemiology
Latent Infection	Persistence of infection in an individual without clinical symptoms and often without detectable test values
Latent Period	Period between exposure to the agent and appearance of disease
Subclinical Disease	Disease that shows no clinical symptoms and must be detected by diagnostic tests only

Related Principles

Modes of transmission
Herd immunity
Screening (Surveillance)

Classic Citation

Sartwell, P.E. 1950. The distribution of incubation period of infectious disease. Am. J. Hygiene 51:310-318. (classic)

References

Burnet, M., and White, D.O. 1972. Natural history of infectious diseases. Cambridge University Press, New York.

Lilienfield, A.M., and Lilienfield, D.E. 1980. Foundations of epidemiology. Second edition. Oxford University Press, New York. Revised by Lilienfield, D.E., and Stolley, P.D. (eds.) 1994. Foundations of epidemiology. Third edition. Oxford University Press, New York.

Mausner, J.S., and Kramer, S. 1985. Mausner and Bahn, Epidemiology: an introductory text. WB Saunders Co. Philadelphia, Pennsylvania.

Modes of Transmission of Disease

Determining the mode of transmission of disease is critical to understanding the epidemiology of the disease, its survival in the population, and methods of control. The distribution of person, place, and time of the disease in the population can help formulate hypotheses about the mode of transmission of disease of an unknown etiology.

Explanation

The transmission of a pathogen is essential for survival of disease in the population and is an important clue to understanding all diseases whether they are infectious or noninfectious. The main categories of the modes of transmission are direct and indirect transmission.

Direct transmission of the disease requires close association or contact between a reservoir of the disease and a susceptible host. Contact with infected skin, mucous membranes, or droplets from an infected human or animal can cause disease. Sexually-transmitted diseases are passed through direct transmission. Droplet spread is differentiated from indirect airborne transmission because the droplets are large particles that travel only a few feet and are often removed by the upper respiratory passages or mucous membranes. Soil or vegetation containing parasites, bacteria, spores, or mycoses may also be a source of direct transmission of disease.

Indirect transmission is more complicated and involves intermediaries that carry the agent of disease from one source to another. The intermediary may be air (airborne), an arthropod (vectorborne), or inanimate object or fomite (vehicleborne through water, food, or blood). Indirect airborne transmission involves spread of the infectious agent through tiny dust or droplet particles over long distances. Particles under 5 microns can be inhaled into the alveoli deep into the lung and are important in environmental and occupational diseases such as asbestosis and silicosis. Food and water are also vehicles of indirect spread and can be a source of localized exposure. Both are sources of bacterial, viral, and parasitic diseases. Water is also known as a source of chemical, environmental, or metal contaminants that can cause serious disease.

Various types of arthropods, such as mosquitoes, ticks, and fleas, are involved as vectors. Each vector has its own life cycle that can often be reflected by seasonal and geographic patterns of transmission of disease. The arthropods can merely carry the agent mechanically to a susceptible host or may be involved biologically in multiplication of the organism or a stage of development. Because vectorborne transmission involves a living organism, the cycle of transmission is often complicated and may involve several levels of maturation of the organism through several reservoirs and hosts. Reservoirs and hosts are differentiated by the fact that reservoirs are essential for the organism's survival and reproduction; hosts supply an environment for the maintenance but not for the survival of an organism. A primary or definitive host is where a parasite achieves maturity or passes through a sexual stage. A secondary or intermediate host usually maintains an organism in a larval or asexual state.

Carriers are individuals that can spread disease either directly or indirectly and are important in the transmission of disease in a population. Carriers are infected individuals with no apparent illness even though they are infected. Depending on the disease involved, the carrier state can be transient or chronic. Obviously, a chronic carrier is more important in the transmission of disease in the population because they

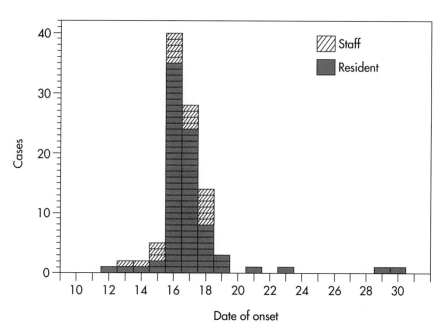

Fig. 2-8 A point-source epidemic curve of an outbreak of influenza in nursing home—Louisiana, August, 1993. (From CDC.1993. Influenza A outbreaks—Louisiana, August 1993. MMWR 42(36):689-692.)

can infect individuals over a long period of time and large geographic areas.

If the mode of transmission is unknown, plotting the number of diseased cases over time may offer some clue to the mode of transmission and to the etiology of disease; these graphs are often called epidemic curves (Fig. 2-8). A curve that has a single peak often reflects a single or localized exposure or infection; this is called a point source. For example, food infected with infectious bacteria at a picnic would cause people at that picnic to become ill. The first outbreak of Legionnaire's disease occurred in a hotel in Philadelphia and showed a point-source curve. Conversely, the epidemic curve can have several increases or peaks over time; this is a propagated epidemic curve (Fig. 2-9). For example, a disease such as influenza that is transmitted from person to person would show a number of increases in disease over time.

Knowledge of the mode of transmission of a disease is essential for the control of that disease in a population. Control programs for directly-transmitted diseases can be aimed at diagnosing and treating carriers, isolating infected individuals, and preventing contact with infected materials. Control of indirectly-transmitted diseases can be

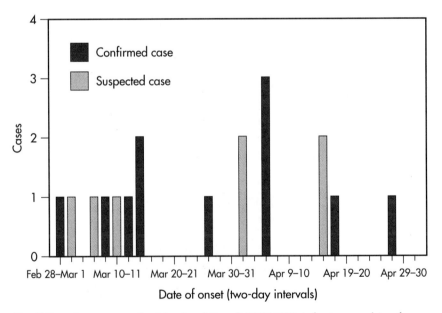

Fig. 2-9 A propagated epidemic of *E. coli* 0104:H21 infection resulting from continued exposure to contaminated milk—Helena, Montana, 1994. (From CDC. 1995. Outbreak of acute gastroenteritis attributable to *Escherichia coli* Serotype 0104:H21—Helena, Montana, 1994. MMWR 44(27):501-504.)

more complicated especially if the mode of transmission is not entirely clear. Airborne transmission over long distances may not be obvious. For those diseases transmitted by known intermediaries, control programs are directed toward the intermediary. Spraying to kill the mosquitoes to control encephalitis outbreaks is an example of a control program.

Example

Lyme disease is the most commonly reported vectorborne disease in the United States and is caused by the spirochete, *Borrelia burgdorferi*. Although several ticks have been found infected with the organism, the deer tick of the *Ixodes* genus is the primary vector. The geographic distribution of Lyme disease correlates with the natural distribution of the Ixodes ticks. Endemic areas are located along the Atlantic coast from Massachusetts south to Georgia, the upper Midwest, and in the West in California and Oregon. However, as recognition of Lyme disease increased, sporadic cases have been reported in most of the states.

TERMS

Arthropod	An invertebrate animal (e.g., insect, arachnid) with jointed body and limbs and usually a chitinous shell that is periodically molted
Host	A living organism that offers an environment for maintenance of an infectious agent.
Intermediate Host(Secondary)	Host where the infectious agent stays at immature or asexual stage
Pathogen	Agent that causes disease
Primary Host (Definitive)	Host where the infectious agent passes through a sexual stage or a maturation process
Reservoir	An inanimate or living organism that is essential for multiplication and therefore survival of an organism
Vector	A living organism that transmits a pathogen. A person with inapparent disease that is infectious to others. Carriers can be temporary, for example, through incubatory and asymptomatic periods or carriers can be chronic

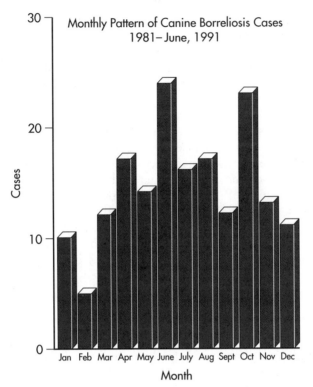

Fig. 2-10 Monthly patterns of canine Lyme disease—1981 to 1991. (From Author's study of Veterinary Medical Database Program involving U.S. veterinary schools [Unpublished]).

Ixodes ticks require at least three hosts for a maturation process that takes 2 years. Each stage of development (larvae, nymph, and adult) is linked to specific hosts or reservoirs, to a specific season, and to the probability of infecting animals or humans. The larvae emerge in late summer to feed on mammals, such as the white-footed mouse, and then remain quiet through the winter. Nymphs develop in the spring to feed on small- and medium-sized mammals, such as mice, squirrels, and opossums. The adult ticks mature on large mammals, such as the white-tailed deer, from late fall to late spring and are less likely to infect humans. The seasonal distribution of the disease cases reported in humans occurs primarily in the summer and fall and correlates with the larval and nymphal stages of the life cycle of the tick and the probability of the humans and animals coming into contact with ticks in the spring and summer months (Fig. 2-10).

Susceptible hosts that have displayed clinical disease are humans, dogs, cattle, and horses. Control of this disease has been directed toward avoiding tick-infested areas and using tick repellents (Fig. 2-11).

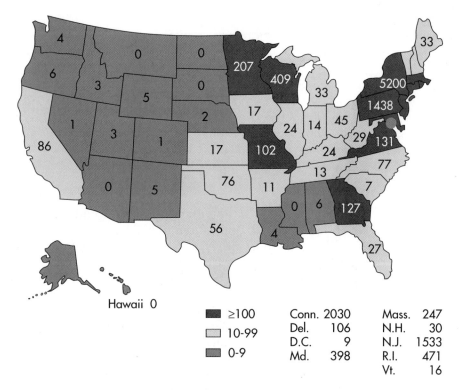

Fig. 2-11   Geographic distribution of Lyme disease cases in the United States, 1994. (From CDC. 1995. Lyme disease—United States, 1994. MMWR 44(24):459-461.)

Related Principles

Person, place, and time
Natural history of disease
Prevention and control (Overview)
Herd immunity
Screening (Surveillance)

References

Benenson, A.S. (ed.) 1995. Control of Communicable Diseases in Man, Sixteenth edition. American Public Health Association, Washington, D.C.

Last, J.M. (ed.) 1984. A dictionary of epidemiology, Second edition. Oxford University Press, New York.

Mausner, J.S., and Kramer, S. 1985. Mausner and Bahn, Epidemiology: an introductory text. WB Saunders Co. Philadelphia, Pennsylvania.

Yorke, J.A., Nathanson, N., Pianigiani, G., and Martin, J. 1979. Seasonality and the requirements for perpetuation and eradication of viruses in populations. Am. J. of Epidemiol. 109(2):103-123.

Herd Immunity

Herd immunity describes the ability to protect susceptible individuals in a group from disease by the presence of a high proportion of immune individuals in the same population. Whether the susceptible individuals are infected depends on how many immune individuals are in the population and how likely the susceptibles are to come into contact with an infected individual. The concept of herd immunity is used to control and prevent disease in populations.

Explanation

Herd immunity is an important concept in understanding the existence of disease in a population, the fluctuation in the number of cases in a population, and even the temporal trends of infectious diseases in a population. Herd immunity is the ability of a proportion of immune individuals in a population to offer some level of protection against infection to the susceptible individuals in a population by decreasing the probability that the susceptibles will come in contact with infected individuals. For herd immunity to be effective, the proportion of immune individuals in a population does not have to be 100%. The proportion of immune individuals in a population depends on the specific disease, the infectivity of the agent, mode of transmission, behavior patterns, and characteristics of the population. Although the exact proportion that needs to be immune to protect the susceptible individuals is still debated, there have been reported ranges of 30% to 70%.

The more important issue is not the percentage of immune individuals but rather the probability of contact of the susceptible individuals with infected individuals. The more frequent and sustained contact the susceptible population has with infected individuals, the more likely the susceptible individuals will become infected and the more likely the disease will remain at high levels in the population. Therefore crowding conditions or small active groups are likely to have increased numbers of cases. Infrequent or short contacts among susceptible and infected individuals will decrease the likelihood of the susceptibles becoming infected and it will keep the disease at a relatively steady, low level. Thus large populations with little interaction among individuals will likely have a small number of cases. Absence of contact, either by isolation of the susceptibles, or dispersal of the population (migration) can end an acute, large increase in the number infected. The dynamics of a population are important to herd immunity.

Knowledge of the herd immunity concept is used in planning a program for disease control and prevention of infectious diseases. One method of prevention is immunization of a proportion of a susceptible population to decrease the number of susceptibles in a population. This is an important method because the entire population does not need to be immunized to control the disease.

Examples

This theory has been used to eliminate smallpox and to reduce polio. Smallpox was eliminated because there was a successful vaccination program. In addition, the disease was easy to diagnose by the lesions on a person's face and skin. Smallpox had a long incubation period, low infectivity, a seasonal pattern, and had a high rate of fatalities. Infected individuals were only infectious for a few days. The seasonal pattern allowed the immunization program to be timed according to the highest period of disease. Smallpox was transmitted directly from person to person so there was no need to control vectors.

Measles is also a good example. Outbreaks of measles usually occur in unvaccinated, preschool-age children and in recent years, college students that previously received only one vaccine. College is a good environment for a large, crowded population of susceptible individuals. In 1990 Milwaukee reported an extensive measles outbreak in preschool children. Vaccination of over 90% of children offers effective protection, but it was not known at the time of the outbreak, what the vaccination coverage was in different subgroups in Milwaukee, particularly the preschool kids. A survey was undertaken to determine vaccination rates. Vaccination rates differed according to race, population density (location), and age. For one census tract, 75% of whites were vaccinated by 2 years of age compared to 62% of Hispanics and 55% of African Americans. The attack rates of measles in census tracts with a higher percentage of African Americans were higher than in census tracts with a lower percentage. (11.3 per 1000 [>50%] versus 2.8 per 1000 [10% to 49%]). In higher population densities, such as the inner cities, the attack rates were higher (6.9 per 1000 [965 people per square kilometer] versus 1.5 per 1000).

There is a high correlation between increasing measles vaccination and decreasing measles transmission. In this study increasing the average immunization rate from 50% to 60% decreased the attack rate from 11.6 to 5.0 per 100. At 81% vaccination, the attack rate was zero.

TERMS

Herd Immunity	The ability of a proportion of immune individuals in a population to protect susceptibles in the population from becoming infected by decreasing the likelihood that the susceptibles come in contact with infected individuals
Outbreak	An increase in the number of individuals with disease, used when talking about infectious diseases

Related Principles
Modes of transmission
Natural history of disease
Epidemic, endemic (Measures of frequency and association)
Prevention and control (Overview)
Population medicine (Overview)

References
Fine, P.E.M. 1993. Herd immunity: history, theory, practice. Epidemiologic Rev. 1993 (15):265-302.
Fox, J.P., Elveback, L., Scott, W., Gatewood, L., and Ackerman, E. 1971. Herd immunity: basic concept and relevance to public health immunization practices. Am. J. of Epidemiol. 94(3):170-189.
Schlenker T.L., Bain C., Baughman A.L., and Hadler S.C. 1992. Measles herd immunity: the association of attack rates with immunization rates in preschool children. JAMA 267(6):823-826.
Topley W.W.C., Wilson G.S. 1923. The spread of bacterial infection. The problem of herd immunity. J. Hyg. 21:243-249.

Epidemiologic Concepts of Disease: Study Questions

1. The Food and Drug Administration (FDA) has requested that healthcare facilities within one state report for the month of December any adverse reactions that occurred within a short time after administration of a particular antibiotic. What is wrong with this definition? What effect will it have on reporting of adverse reactions? How would you state the case definition? What conclusions will the FDA be able to make? How would you design a study to look at possible side effects resulting from a particular antibiotic in a hospital setting?

2. Describe the possible etiology of a disease that is occurring in lumberjacks and foresters in Washington, Oregon, and California and is occurring most often during the spring and summer months. Select and describe one infectious and one chronic disease that exhibits age effects, has a temporal trend, and has a geographic pattern.

3. Give an example of a disease for each of the types of transmission and describe how the descriptive epidemiology relates to the transmission mode. Explain the control and prevention methods for each disease and how they relate to the transmission of the disease.

4. Why would determining if there is a difference between generation period and incubation period be important if you were trying to stop the spread of an infectious disease within a closed population?

5. Explain the importance of a disease with a long subclinical phase in implementing a surveillance program to determine the number of cases of disease and in implementing a control program for the disease.

6. Explain how herd immunity is affected by a population that is closed (no movement of people in or out) versus a dynamic population (people coming in and out).

7. Research the eradication program of smallpox. Why was this campaign successful although the campaign to eliminate tuberculosis was not?

8. Give an example of a disease that would be reflected by a point source epidemic curve and a disease that would be reflected by a propagated epidemic curve. Why?

9. Explain the importance of carriers in the transmission of disease.

10. Give two examples of diseases that are affected by herd immunity in the population.

11. What is wrong with the assumption that an increase in secular trends is due to an increase in the disease of interest?

12. Describe the characteristics related to people that are important in the study of epidemiology. Give an example of a disease that is influenced by each, for example, age.

13. Why is age such an important consideration in the epidemiology of a disease?

CHAPTER 3

Measures of Frequency and Association

Measurements of the proportion of a population with a particular characteristic are quoted daily by politicians, the news media, and scientists. These numbers give valuable information to the general public. Likewise, measurements of the frequency of a disease or an event occurring in a population give important information to epidemiologists. By measuring the proportion of persons affected and describing the distribution of affected individuals by region and time, epidemiologists are given important descriptive epidemiologic information. This information aids in determining the etiology and possible risk factors of a disease.

Measures of frequency for each group or population can be used to make comparisons among groups and to estimate the likelihood that a particular exposure or risk factor is associated with a disease. By comparing groups with different characteristics, the associations of different risk factors related to a disease can be explored. The measures of **Rate, Ratio,** or **Proportion,** begin in simple mathematic terms with a **Numerator** and a **Denominator.** The numerator represents the number of cases, events, or characteristics of interest, and the denominator represents the number in the group being studied. A rate, ratio, or proportion measurement of the frequency of disease is essential in the understanding of the distribution of a disease in a population, in the calculating of the association of possible risk factors for a disease, and in the studying of the epidemiology of a disease.

Understanding what the numerator and denominator represent in the measurement of a disease or event over time enables epidemiologists to estimate the **Incidence** and **Prevalence.** These measures of frequency can help estimate the risk or the probability of a member of a group or population becoming ill or diseased over time. By measuring the rate of disease or the number of cases or events over time in a geographic region, an estimate of whether a disease is **Epidemic** or **Endemic** can be made. The occurrence of an epidemic initiates immediate public health action.

Once measures are used to determine the distribution or frequency of attributes, the real challenge of epidemiology is to try to determine the cause of or the risk factors for a disease. **Relative Risk** or **Odds Ratio** is used as measure of comparison of two groups or populations. By comparing groups or populations differing in exposures or demographics, these measures estimate the association between different exposures or risk factors and a disease; consequently, groups with different exposures or risk factors have a different risk or probability of getting a disease. Relative risk and odds ratio measurements estimate the association of exposure and disease and the risk of a member of a population for getting the disease given the exposure.

Attributable Risk, by comparing the differences in risk between two groups, measures the magnitude of the effect of the exposure on the frequency of disease in the groups. It is important to realize that to compare two or more groups they must be as similar as possible with the exception of the factor being analyzed, otherwise the results of the comparisons are unclear. **Standardization** of the rates is one method to make comparisons among groups possible.

List of Principles

Rates, Ratios, Proportions
Rates measure the change in an event over time in a population that is at risk. Rates are the most accurate measure of risk because they measure a population without disease but at risk for a disease in the beginning of a time period and the rate of disease that occurs during the time period. Ratios are used when it is difficult to define the total population at risk. Ratios do not measure the change over time and are used as summary measures and approximations of risk. It is important in the conclusions made about the measures to know whether the measure is a rate or ratio.

Numerator, Denominator
To make accurate conclusions about the distribution of disease in a population, it is important to define the numerator and the denominator. This includes knowing whether one or both numbers also measure time. It also involves determining whether the numerator measures cases or events and determining what population the denominator represents.

Incidence, Prevalence	Incidence represents the rate of occurrence of new cases of disease or an event in a population at risk during a specified period of time. Prevalence represents the number of existing cases of disease at a given point in time. Because incidence measures the rate of change of disease or an event, it can be used to express the risk of becoming ill. Prevalence can only estimate the probability of the population being ill at a period of time studied. If incident cases continue to remain diseased over time, then they become prevalent cases; therefore prevalence equals incidence times duration.
Epidemic, Endemic	If the number of cases of a disease in a region remains relatively stable over a long period of time, the disease is considered to be endemic in the area. If the number increases greatly over the expected or normal level, then there is an epidemic of that disease. No specific number is used to determine when there is an epidemic; it varies with the disease and the usual number of cases.
Relative Risk	The comparison of the incidence rates of disease for two populations, one with a factor of interest, one without, estimates the association of that factor and the disease. The value of the relative risk represents the strength of the association. An association between a factor of interest and a disease does not prove that the risk factor causes the disease.
Odds Ratio	The odds ratio is also a measure of the association of a risk factor with disease but is calculated by comparing the odds of exposure for the two populations. Because the incidence of disease is unknown, the absolute risk cannot be calculated, only estimated. However, if the disease is rare, the odds ratio is a good approximation of the relative risk.
Attributable Risk	Attributable risk is a measure of the absolute difference in incidence rates between a group that is exposed to a factor of interest and the incidence rate of a group not exposed. This difference determines how much greater the frequency of disease is in the exposed group than the unexposed group and quantifies the risk attributed to the exposure. One assumption with this measurement is that there is a cause and effect between exposure and disease.

Standardization Populations that differ significantly in an important host factor or attribute, such as age, which may affect disease, cannot be accurately compared. Instead the two groups that are to be compared must be "adjusted" or standardized for that factor. Standardization is done by calculating hypothetic rates for each group according to an artificial distribution of that factor that is comparable for both groups.

Rates, Ratios, Proportions

Rates measure the change in an event over time in a population that is at risk. Rates are the most accurate measure of risk because they measure a population without disease but at risk for a disease in the beginning of a time period and the rate of disease that occurs during the time period. Ratios are used when it is difficult to define the total population at risk. Ratios do not measure the change over time and are used as summary measures and approximations of risk. It is important in the conclusions made about the measures to know whether the measure is a rate or ratio.

Explanation

The actual definitions for rates, ratios, and proportions involve simple mathematics, but it is important to understand the differences among the measurements. A part of what differentiates the three measurements is what the numerator and denominator represent. If proper conclusions about the measurement are to be made, it is vital to understand the differences in what the rate, ratio, and proportion represent.

A proportion consists of a numerator that is always part of the denominator and is expressed as a percentage. Rates and ratios are considered forms of a proportion. Proportions are common measurements used in surveys or polls of a population and are easy to estimate because no time period is needed. However, the useful information is limited. If a time period is specified and the denominator is the population at risk, the proportion becomes a rate.

A rate measures the occurrence of a disease or the number of a particular characteristic or event during a period of time in a population at risk. The items being counted in the numerator represent the number of cases or events that occur in the denominator or the population at risk during a specified period of time. In other words, a rate is:

x cases/y people per unit of time

The population in the denominator is the population at the beginning of the specified time period that is at risk for getting the disease or event of interest. At the end of the specified time period, there are the individuals that developed the disease or the event (numerator) and individuals that did not. A rate measures the rate of change over time of the disease or event. Because the rate starts at the beginning of a time period with a population at risk but without disease and ends at a time with actual cases of diseases, it is possible to calculate the probability or risk of the population developing the disease at the beginning of a time period.

In some situations, it is difficult to define the total population at risk for a disease. A common alternative taken is to use the ratio of the number of cases or events that have occurred in a calculated number of the population as a measure of frequency of the disease or event in a population (diseased/nondiseased). A ratio consists of a numerator that may not be a part of the population at risk (denominator) and the denominator may not be the population at risk. For example, a comparison of women (numerator) and men (denominator) diagnosed with malignant melanoma does not have a numerator that is part of the denominator or a denominator that is the population at risk. The denominator is more likely a sample of the population. In the purest sense, x and y are independent of each other (x/y). A ratio does not measure the rate of change over time and the risk of developing of disease. However, ratios are used as a summary measure and an approximation of risk.

The term *rate* is often mistakenly used when discussing a ratio. These should not be considered equivalent when making conclusions about the risk of disease. In epidemiology, ratios and even proportions are used to describe the distribution of person, place, and time and the occurrence of disease in a population. A rate measures change of time in disease and the probability of developing that disease in a population. According to Elandt-Johnson in 1975, "ratios are indices, proportions are relative frequencies and can estimate probabilities of certain events, while rates describe the speed and direction of change."

Example

Abortion ratio versus abortion rate:

> Abortion ratio equals the number of legal induced abortions/1000 live births
> Abortion rate equals the number of legal induced abortions/1000 women, ages 15 to 44 years, per year. (The ages of 15 to 44 are the usual time period of child-bearing although there are extremes.)

In the United States the abortion ratio in 1987 was 356/1000 although the abortion rate was 24/1000. The denominator in the abor-

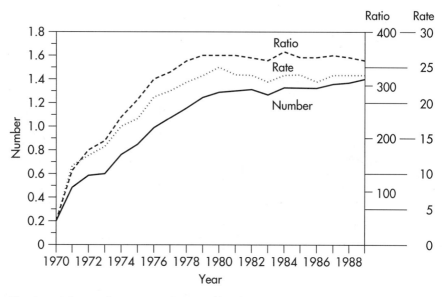

Fig. 3-1 The number, rate, and ratio of legal abortions in the United States, by year, 1970 to 1989.
Number = in millions.
Rate = per 1,000 women from ages 15 to 44 years.
Ratio = per 1,000 live births.
(From Koonin, L.M., Smith, J.C., Ramick, M., and Lawson, H.W. Abortion Surveillance—United States, 1989. In: CDC Surveillance Summaries, September, 1992. MMWR 1992; 41(SS-5):1-9.)

tion ratio does not take into consideration stillbirths or miscarriages. The abortion rate denominator takes into consideration the true population at risk.

Fig. 3-1 shows the difference in the information represented by a rate and a ratio. It is important to know what is being measured.

TERMS

Proportion	A special form of a ratio where the numerator is part of the denominator
Rate	A measure of frequency of a disease or event in a population that always includes time. It measures the change of an event over time
Ratio	Consists of a numerator and denominator that are usually independent of each other

Related Principles
Numerator, denominator
Incidence, prevalence

Classic Citation
Fleiss, J.L. 1991. Statistical methods for rates and proportions. Second edition. John Wiley & Sons, New York.

References
CDC, Epidemiology Program Office, Public Health Practice Program Office, DHHS. 1992. Principles of epidemiology, Second Edition. Self-study course 3030-G. Atlanta, Georgia.

Elandt-Johnson, R.C. 1975. Definition of rates: some remarks on their use and misuse. Am. J. Epidemiol. 102:267-271.

Koonin, L.M., Smith, J.C., Ramick, M., and Lawson, H.W. 1992. Abortion Surveillance United States, 1989. In: CDC Surveillance Summaries, September, 1992. MMWR 41(SS-5):1-9.

Roht, L.H., Selwyn, B.J., Holguin, A.H., and Christensen, B.L. 1982. Principles of epidemiology: a self-teaching guide. Academic Press. Orlando, Florida. Chapters 2 and 3.

Numerator and Denominator

To make accurate conclusions about the distribution of disease in a population, it is important to define the numerator and the denominator. This includes knowing whether one or both numbers also measure time. It also involves determining whether the numerator measures cases or events and determining what population the denominator represents.

Explanation

Commercials or the news media often use statements such as, "1 out of 4 use aspirin." But what does this mean? One of the first questions to ask is what does the 1 and the 4 represent. Both the numerator and denominator need to be understood before accurate conclusions about a measurement are made.

The numerator, or the top number in a fraction (x/y), measures the number of x. This may be the number of cases of a disease, the number of deaths, or the number of events, such as adverse drug reactions. It is important to know what the numerator measures and what the definition for that measurement is. Depending on the event being measured, one person may be counted only once or several times. For example, a person can die only once but the same individual could experience multiple adverse drug reactions. Similarly, the numerator that includes only the new cases of a disease is different from a numerator that counts all of the existing cases of a disease. In general, unless a disease is rapidly fatal, the number of existing cases is larger than the number of new cases. The number of existing cases of disease would be affected by any factor that would affect a disease over time. The number of new cases over time would allow the calculation of the rate of change of a disease over time. Consequently, the risk to a population for developing that particular disease or event can be calculated.

In understanding any measurement, the denominator is often the most difficult to define and measure. One of the most important questions to answer is whether the denominator represents the *total* population under study or at risk for a disease or an event, or just a sample of the population. Ideally, the denominator should be a measure of the population truly at risk for an event of interest. For example, when calculating the birth rate in a population, including all women in the denominator would not be accurate because not all women are able to give birth (e.g., very young girls; women with hysterectomies, menopause). The rate would be artificially low because the denominator would be inaccurately high. Instead, birth rate is generally calculated using the number of women, ages 15 to 44 years, in the population as the denominator. This would be the population at risk of having births and would yield a more representative denominator and rate. The more representative the denominator is of the true population, the more accurate the conclusions.

To calculate a rate, the denominator must consider not only the total population at risk but also the amount of time that each individual in that population is at risk. The calculation of person-time units of exposure is included in the denominator. A person, for example, may be exposed for 6 months while another person is exposed for 14 months. If the population is large and if the number remains steady in that population, then it is appropriate that the denominator be estimated by the average population at a midpoint in the time period. For example, a commonly used denominator is the population at the midpoint of the year. In other words, it is assumed that everyone in the midyear population has had a year of exposure. The problem with this denominator is that it assumes that all individuals are present and at risk for the same period of time. If the population under study is small, resulting in a lot of movement of individuals in and out of the total population and a wide variation in exposure time, then a more precise measurement is needed. The calculation of the actual person-time units of exposure gives a more precise denominator. The exposure time for each individual is calculated and summed with the other individuals in the denominator.

Using person-time units in the denominator assumes that the risk is constant over time and that all of the individuals are similar with regard to the disease rate. Despite those assumptions, person-time units are precise and enable comparisons among groups because the units are equivalent and independent.

By changing the numerator or denominator, the specific type of ratio, rate, or proportion needed can be calculated. All that is essential is to know what is measured. For example, a mortality rate for a particular disease is the number of deaths resulting from a particular disease (numerator) divided by the number of population at risk (denominator). The case-fatality rate measures the severity of a disease by calculating the number of deaths caused by a disease (numerator) divided by the total number of cases of the disease or population at risk (denominator).

Examples

1. A subdivision in West Virginia has a total of 5 households that contain a total of 9 people. When these people were interviewed, 4 of the 9 people reported having a headache during the month of December. Three of these four reported having at least four headaches during December. The rate of occurrence of headaches per population is different than the number of headaches per population.

   Number of headaches/population equals 13/9.

   Number of people who develop headaches equals 4/9.

   What information do you really want?

2. In a population of 500 government workers, we want to calculate the proportion that missed at least 2 days of work during the month of September. Of those 500 workers, 5 were on sick leave for the entire month. Of the remaining 495 workers, 25 missed at least 2 days of work.

   a. A crude measure is the number of people who missed at least 2 days divided by the total population.

   $$30/500 = 6 \text{ per } 100$$

   b. A more precise measure would take into consideration the actual time of exposure. This would require eliminating those workers on sick leave. These five workers are not at risk. The time period in which the population can miss a working day in a month is actually 20 working days (5 working days/week). It does not include weekends. This is 10,000 working days. Therefore 25 ($\times$ 2 days)/(500 – 5) times 20 working days equals 50/9900 equals 5.1 per 1000 person-working days. This is an accurate rate that enables the calculation of the probability or risk of missing a work day. Ideally, it would be important to know how many days each of those 25 individuals missed to calculate the most accurate measurement.

TERMS

Case-Fatality Rate	The proportion of the cases with a certain disease that results in death in a certain time period
Morbidity Rate	The proportion of the population that becomes ill during a period of time
Mortality Rate	The proportion of a population that dies during a period of time

Related Principles
Case definition (Epidemiologic concepts of disease)
Person, place, time (Epidemiologic concepts of disease)
Epidemic, endemic
Incidence, prevalence
Rate, ratio, proportion

References
Mausner J.S. and Kramer S. 1985. Mausner and Bahn: Epidemiology: an introductory text. W.B. Saunders Company. Philadelphia, Pennsylvania.
Roht, L.H., Selwyn, B.J., Holguin, A.H., and Christensen, B.L. 1982. Principles of epidemiology: a self-teaching guide. Academic Press. Orlando, Florida. Chapters 2 and 3.

Incidence and Prevalence

Incidence represents the rate of occurrence of new cases of disease or an event in a population at risk during a specified period of time. Prevalence represents the number of existing cases of disease at a given point in time. Because incidence measures the rate of change of disease or an event, it can be used to express the risk of becoming ill. Prevalence can only estimate the probability of the population being ill at a period of time studied. If incident cases continue to remain diseased over time, then they become prevalent cases; therefore prevalence equals incidence times duration.

Explanation

It is important to differentiate between the incidence and prevalence of a disease so that correct conclusions about the disease can be made. The incidence rate is the most direct method of calculating risk. The numerator in the incidence rate is the number of new cases that occur during a specific period of time. The denominator is the sum of total amount of time during which any individual in the population was at risk. The incidence rate measures the frequency with which new cases occur in the population and expresses the risk or probability of illness in a population over a period of time.

The term *attack rate* is often used instead of the incidence rate in infectious diseases or during an outbreak of disease in a narrowly defined population over a short period of time. The attack rate is calculated as the number affected divided by the number exposed and can be useful in determining the source of an infection. For example, in the case of a food-borne outbreak, the attack rate can be calculated for different types of foods eaten. The attack rates for the different types of foods can be compared to find the food that is causing the illness. In outbreaks resulting from an individual source, the index case in an outbreak is the first case reported. The secondary attack rate is the frequency of new cases among the population that occur after the first case. It is calculated with the first or index case excluded from the numerator and denominator. The secondary attack rate indicates the degree of infectivity and communicability of the disease. A high secondary attack rate, or a large number of infected people per exposure, indicates high infectivity. In other words, a large number of people became infected with little exposure.

Prevalence represents the number of existing cases of disease or events at a certain time period. It focuses on whether a disease is present or not, rather than whether the disease is a new case. Prevalence is less precise than incidence and is not focused on time. It is important to determine the earliest onset of illness; otherwise, actual incident cases will be classified incorrectly as prevalent cases. Prevalence measures disease status in a "snapshot" in time rather than from the time of onset of disease. The denominator of a prevalence measure is the general population, not necessarily the population at risk. Although the term *prevalence rate* is often used in journals, prevalence is actually a ratio.

Because prevalence measures only existing cases of disease, it is more useful in the study of chronic than acute diseases. The duration of illness of chronic diseases is long; therefore prevalence can be measured at any time and still capture the number of individuals that is chronically ill. The more likely an individual is to survive with a chronic disease, the higher the prevalence value. Chronic diseases that have a large percentage of rapid deaths would have fewer individuals who remained chronically ill and be included in a prevalence measurement. Prevalence, therefore, not only measures the risk factors of disease but also those factors that influence the survival of an individual with the disease. The probability of having disease at a certain point in time can be calculated even though the risk of becoming ill cannot be calculated. The risk of becoming ill can only be calculated with an incidence rate.

The time period that is chosen for prevalence is arbitrary. Two types of measurements often seen are point prevalence and period prevalence. Point prevalence is the number of existing cases at a specific point in time. For instance, a yearly census exemplifies point prevalence. Period prevalence is the number of cases for a longer, but still limited, period of time. A period prevalence may cover a month or even a year.

Time is an important variable that differentiates incidence and prevalence. Time also can interrelate the two measures by the relationship of prevalence equals incidence times duration (P = I ¥ D). If newly occurring cases (incidence) are not treated and do not die quickly, these cases of disease become existing cases (prevalence); therefore the longer the duration of disease, the more likely that incident cases become prevalent cases and are measured as such. This is an important concept when looking at changes in prevalence of a disease and determining that an increase in the prevalence could either be new cases that have been treated and survive longer or an actual increase in the disease incidence. Diseases with a high incidence may still have an unexpectedly low prevalence if the duration decreases because of fatality or quick recovery.

Example

Two surveys are done one year apart on a small town to look for individuals with high cholesterol (>300) to recruit for a research program. There are 2000 people in this small town, both at the initial and follow-up surveys, and the population remains the same. The initial survey reveals there are 150 people with high cholesterol that remains at a high level. At the time of the second survey, there are a total of 300 with high cholesterol.

The point prevalence at the time of the first survey is:

150/2000 = 0.075 or 75 per 1000

The period prevalence for one year is:

300/2000 × 1000 = 150 per 1000

The incidence, or the number of new cases, during that one year is:

300 − 150 = 150

The actual population at risk is:

2000 − 150 = 1850

(There were 150 existing cases that should be removed from the population at risk).

Therefore the incidence rate (IR) is:

$$150/1850 \times 1000 = 81 \text{ per } 1000$$

TERMS

Attack Rate	A specialized term used for the incidence rate in an epidemic of an infectious disease among susceptibles
Incidence	The number of *new* cases occurring in a given period of time in a population
Period Prevalence	The number of people with disease during a specified time period
Point Prevalence	The number of people with a disease at a point in time
Prevalence	The number of existing cases occurring in a population

Related Principles
Numerator, denominator
Rates, ratios, proportions
Case definition (Epidemiologic concepts of disease)

References
Ahlbom, A., Norell, S. 1984. Introduction to modern epidemiology. Epidemiology Resources. Chestnut Hill, Massachusetts.

Freeman, J., and Hutchinson, G.B. 1980. Prevalence, incidence, and duration. Am. J. Epidemiol. 112:707-723.

Morgenstern, H., Kleinbaum, D.G., and Kupper, L.L. 1980. Measures of disease incidence used in epidemiologic research. Int. J. Epidemiol. 9:97-104.

Roht, L.H., Selwyn B.J., Holguin, A.H., and Christensen, B.L. 1982. Principles of epidemiology: a self-teaching guide. Academic Press. Orlando, Florida.

Rothman, K.J. 1986. Modern epidemiology. Little, Brown and Company. Boston, Massachussetts.

Epidemic, Endemic

If the number of cases of a disease in a region remains relatively stable over a long period of time, the disease is considered to be endemic in the area. If the number increases greatly over the expected or normal level, then there is an epidemic of that disease. No specific number is used to determine when there is an epidemic; it varies with the disease and the usual number of cases.

Explanation

An epidemic occurs when there is an increase over normal in the number of cases of disease in a geographic region or in a period of time. An epidemic can cover any time period; it may be a few weeks or even a few years. A worldwide epidemic is called a pandemic. An epidemic may be an increase in the number of cases of a disease, or it may be an increase in the number of events. The term *outbreak* is also used to refer to an epidemic but is more commonly used to refer to an epidemic that occurs in infectious diseases.

Unfortunately, there is no standardized definition for what is considered an epidemic increase over the normal or expected number. The level of disease or event that is considered at an epidemic level varies with the disease or event and the circumstances. For example, if a disease is very rare or has been eradicated in the United States, then one or two cases of that disease would constitute an epidemic. However, in a different country where the disease is common, one or two cases would not be an epidemic. Determining when an epidemic is occurring is difficult if the normal level of disease in a population is unknown. Active efforts must be made by health departments to determine the rate of a disease in a population if there is a concern.

An endemic disease in a given area is one that has remained at a relatively constant number of cases over a long period of time. A disease is still endemic to an area, though it may occasionally have sporadic increases that can be considered epidemic. A disease that remains epidemic for years with little changes in frequency may be considered endemic. There are also some circumstances where a disease may be epidemic and endemic depending on the geographic area that is being considered.

Examples

1. If a disease is very rare, even one case would be an epidemic (e.g., smallpox). On the other hand, 50 cases of influenza in the middle of the flu season would not be an epidemic.
2. Raccoon rabies is considered endemic in the southeastern United States (e.g., Florida, Georgia). However, when rabies cases began occurring in the Mid-Atlantic states of Virginia, West Virginia, and

Maryland, rabies was considered an epidemic. It is still considered epidemic in New Jersey and New York but is considered endemic in Virginia, Maryland, Pennsylvania, and West Virginia because rabies has remained at fairly stable, though high, levels for several years.

TERMS

Endemic	A constant or steady level of disease in a certain geographic area or population
Epidemic	An increase over the normal and expected level of disease in a given area or population and time period
Epizootic	Term sometimes used instead of epidemic to describe an epidemic disease occurring in animals (e.g., rabies)
Outbreak	Synonym for epidemic, often used in infectious diseases or for a localized epidemic
Pandemic	An epidemic that occurs over a large geographic area (e.g., world) or involves a large proportion of the population

Related Principles
Numerator, denominator
Incidence, prevalence
Person, place, time (Epidemiologic concepts of disease)

References
Last, J.M. (ed). 1988. A dictionary of epidemiology, Second edition. Oxford University Press, New York.
Mausner, J.S., and Kramer, S. 1985. Mausner and Bahn, Epidemiology: an introductory text. W.B. Saunders Co. Philadelphia, Pennsylvania.

Relative Risk

The comparison of the incidence rates of disease for two populations, one with a factor of interest, one without, estimates the association of that factor and the disease. The value of the relative risk represents the strength of the association. An association between a factor of interest and a disease does not prove that the risk factor causes the disease.

Explanation

Incidence and prevalence measures are used to calculate the risk of an individual or a population becoming ill or having a disease or characteristic of interest. The natural consequence of knowing the risk of a disease or an event is to wonder about the factors that might influence that risk. Comparisons of rates or risk of disease between populations that vary in the factor of interest can estimate the association of the factor of interest and the disease or event. The compared populations may differ in demographic factors that might affect a particular disease or event or differ in an a particular exposure of interest. The measure of association between the risk factor and disease is an estimate of risk.

The most precise estimate for comparison is relative risk. Relative risk is the ratio of the incidence rates (or sometimes the estimated risk) of two populations. If the event is a disease, then the relative risk is the incidence rate in the one population with the characteristic of interest or exposure divided by the incidence rate of the other population without the characteristic of interest or exposure. The population of interest is always in the numerator. The calculation of the relative risk is often done by a 2 × 2 table that allows the epidemiologist to organize the risk factor and the disease into groups (diseased and nondiseased, exposed and unexposed) and compare them (see the first example on p. 58). The form and notation of the 2 × 2 table is standard.

This calculation measures the risk of the exposed group relative to the unexposed or how much more likely the exposed group is to become ill than the unexposed group. Obviously, a relative risk of 1.0 means the risk in both groups is identical. There is disagreement among epidemiologists as to what is the "magical" number that shows an increase in relative risk. A risk greater than 1.0 means the exposed group is at increased risk, and a risk of less than 1.0 is interpreted as the exposed group is at less risk. Most epidemiologists would agree that a relative risk of over 2.0 indicates a true increased risk.

Comparing two groups that are exposed or not exposed to a characteristic of interest, results in an estimate of an association between that factor and the disease that develops. The relative risk value gives an estimate of the strength of that association. For example, if the relative risk for the exposed group is 3.5 compared to the unexposed group, then there is a strong association between the exposure and the risk of developing the disease. This is important information that will point epidemiologists toward the study of this possible risk factor to determine if the exposure actually causes the disease. It is important, moreover, to remember that an association between a risk factor and a disease does not necessarily mean that the risk factor causes the disease.

Examples

1.

DISEASE INCIDENCE

Risk Factor	Yes	No	TOTAL AT RISK
Yes	a	b	a + b
No	c	d	c + d
TOTAL	a + c	b + d	

Risk of disease in exposed group equals a/(a + b)
Risk of disease in unexposed group equals c/(c + d)

Relative risk equals a/(a + b) divided by c/(c + d)
a = number of persons with disease and with exposure.
b = number of persons without disease, but with exposure.
c = number of persons with disease, but without exposure.
d = number of persons without disease and without exposure.
a + c = total number of persons with disease.
b + d = total number of persons without disease.

2. A study was done of a population, ages 25 to 45 years, to estimate the risk of being diagnosed with rheumatoid arthritis. There were 3870 people in the population. Of these 3870, 1850 were female and 2020 were male.(Fictional data created for this example.)

DISEASE

Gender	Yes	No	Total
Female	50	1800	1850
Male	20	2000	2020
Total	70	3800	3870

Risk of illness in females is: 50/1850 = 0.027
Risk of illness in males is: 20/2020 = 0.010

Relative risk for illness in females as compared to males is: 2.7/1.0 = 2.7. In this population, females are 2.7 times more likely to have rheumatoid arthritis than males.

TERMS

Exposed	A group that has the characteristic of interest
Relative Risk	The ratio of the incidence rate of disease in an exposed group to the incidence rate of disease in an unexposed group
Unexposed	A group that is without the characteristic of interest

Related Principles

Rates, ratios, proportions
Incidence, prevalence
Prospective, cohort studies (Observational studies)

References

CDC, Epidemiology Program Office, Public Health Practice Program
Office, DHHS. 1992. Principles of epidemiology, Second edition. Self-
study course 3030-G. Atlanta, Georgia.

Hennekens, C.H., Buring, J. and edited by S.L. Mayrent. 1987. Epidemiology in medicine. Little, Brown, and Company. Boston, Massachussetts.

Kahn, H.A., and Sempos, C.T. 1989. Statistical methods in epidemiology. Monographs in epidemiology and biostatistics, Vol 12. Oxford
University Press, New York.

Odds Ratio

*The odds ratio is also a measure of the association of a risk factor with
disease but is calculated by comparing the odds of exposure for the
two populations. Because the incidence of disease is unknown, the
absolute risk cannot be calculated, only estimated. However, if the disease is rare, the odds ratio is a good approximation of the relative risk.*

Explanation

The odds ratio is similar to relative risk in that it is also a measure
of association between a factor of interest and a disease. It can be calculated by using the same 2 × 2 table that is used in the calculation of
the relative risk. The odds ratio is the calculation of the "odds" of having a disease in a population with the characteristic of interest; this is
estimated by comparing a diseased population with the factor of interest
with a population without the disease. The odds ratio is used as an estimate of the relative risk when the incidence rate of disease in an exposed
or unexposed population cannot be calculated. The odds ratio can be
calculated if the prevalence of disease in an exposed and unexposed population is known. It is a particularly good estimate of the relative risk
when a disease is rare. For the odds ratio to be a good approximation,
the cases and controls have to be representative of the general population with respect to the exposure.

The advantages of the odds ratio are the same as using prevalence
instead of incidence. The odds ratio is not affected by factors that influence survival of an individual because the time of onset of disease is not

important. The odds ratio can be used as a measure of association between a factor and disease in more types of study designs and in circumstances in which there is less known about the population. Another advantage is that the odds ratio can be calculated from a 2 × 2 table even if the true size of the population for the cases is unknown. It is not important to know the size of the exposed or the unexposed group. The odds ratio is an easier measure to calculate to give some estimate of risk. This is important when incidence rates are less frequently known.

Examples

RISK FACTOR	CASES	CONTROLS	TOTAL
Yes	a	b	a + b
No	c	d	c + d
Total	a + c	b + d	

Odds of risk factor in cases equals a/c
Odds of risk factor in noncases (or controls) equals b/d

$$\frac{a/c}{b/d} \quad \text{or} \quad ad/bc$$

a/c gives an estimate (odds) of how the cases are divided between those with and without the risk factor and b/d (odds) gives an estimation of the distribution of the risk factor in the noncases.

Using the same disease example from the relative risk concept (p. 58):

DISEASE

Gender	Yes	No	Total
Female	50	1800	1850
Male	20	2000	2020
Total	70	3800	3870

Odds ratio (OR) equals $(50 \times 2000)/(1800 \times 20) = 2.77$

2. Example of how relative risk (RR) equals odds ratio (OR)

$$RR = \frac{a/(a + b)}{c/(c + d)}$$

If the disease is rare then,
a (cases with disease and risk factor) is small compared to b and a/(a + b) approximates a/b and
c (cases with disease without risk factor) is small compared to d and c/(c + d) approximates c/d

and . . . .

$$\frac{a/b}{c/d} \quad \text{or} \quad ad/bc$$

OR equals

$$\frac{a/c}{b/d} \quad \text{or} \quad ad/bc$$

TERMS

Odds Ratio   The ratio of the odds of getting the disease in the exposed over the odds of getting the disease in the unexposed. Also called the cross-products ratio

Related Principles
Relative risk
Incidence, prevalence
Case-control, retrospective studies (Observational studies)

References
Cornfield, J. 1951. A method of estimating comparative rates from clinical data: applications to cancer of the lung, breast, and cervix. Journal of National Cancer Institute 11:1269-1275.
Kahn, H.A., and Sempos, C.T. 1989. Statistical methods in epidemiology. Monographs in epidemiology and biostatistics, Vol 12. Oxford University Press, New York.
Schlesselman, J.J. 1982. Case-control studies: design, conduct, analysis. Monographs in epidemiology and biostatistics, Vol 2. Oxford University Press. New York.

Attributable Risk

Attributable risk is a measure of the absolute difference in incidence rates between a group that is exposed to a factor of interest and the incidence rate of a group not exposed. This difference determines how much greater the frequency of disease is in the exposed group than the unexposed group and quantifies the risk attributed to the exposure. One assumption with this measurement is that there is a cause and effect between exposure and disease.

Explanation

In contrast to the relative risk and odds ratio that compared the likelihoods of becoming ill for two groups, the attributable risk (AR) calculates how much greater the frequency of disease is in the exposed group. By looking at the differences in rates rather than a ratio of rates, AR measures the absolute effect of the exposure on the frequency of disease. Consequently, it is possible to estimate the amount of illness that could be prevented by eliminating the factor or exposure. An estimate is useful for the determination of whether a program aimed at elimination or control of that risk factor is worthwhile. Comparison of this information for several diseases can help public health practitioners determine which diseases are of the greatest public health importance. It is more beneficial to initiate a program to control a risk factor that has a large effect on the frequency of a disease than to control a risk factor that has little effect. This is especially true if the particular disease affects a large number of people. This is important information for public health decisions and to determine public health impact of a prevention or control program.

There are several terms used for this general concept such as attributable risk, population attributable risk, etiologic fraction, attributable fraction, and attributable risk percent (attributable proportion). Each term can be interpreted slightly differently yet they are often used interchangeably. For accuracy and clarity, it is important to determine precisely what is measured.

Attributable risk can be calculated for a single group or for a total population (population attributable risk). One assumption hidden in the formula that helps in understanding AR is that exposure to a specific risk factor accounts for only a portion of the incidence rate in the exposed group. The incidence rate of the exposed is actually the sum of the incidence rate *not* due to exposure and the incidence rate due to exposure. Consequently, when the incidence rate of the unexposed is subtracted from the incidence rate of the exposed, the number remaining is how much of the disease is due to the exposure. Attributable risk equals incidence exposed minus incidence unexposed. The attributable risk percentage is simply:

Incidence rate exposed − Incidence rate unexposed/Incidence rate exposed × 100

This is the percentage of a person's risk for disease that is caused by the exposure; consequently, by extension it is how much disease can be prevented by elimination of that exposure.

The attributable risk for a population or population attributable risk (PAR) measures the proportion of total cases of a disease that are associated with a risk factor in the total population. This can be used to estimate the diseases most important to the community. Because PAR relates to the total population, both the relative risk and the population prevalence are important in the formula. The population attributable risk is:

Incidence rate (total population) – Incidence rate (unexposed) or
AR multiplied by the P(exp) [proportion of exposed individuals in the population].

The population attributable risk originated from Levin (1953), and the formula used most often, especially if the incidence rates are unknown, is called Levin's formula:

$$\frac{p(rr-1)}{p(rr-1)+1}$$

p= Prevalence of risk factor in the population
r= Relative risk

OR

$$\frac{\text{Incidence in total population} - \text{incidence in unexposed}}{\text{Incidence in total population}}$$

In this formula, as prevalence of the risk factor increases, PAR increases, and it more closely approximates AR percentage. The attributable risk of the exposed is almost always greater than PAR because the effect of eliminating the exposure from the number of cases is greater than from the general population that is composed of exposed and unexposed. So, if an exposure is extremely rare, even if it is strongly related to the disease, PAR will still be small. Conversely, a common exposure will have a large PAR.

The population attributable risk is important in measuring the public health impact of the factor and for making public health policy decisions. The population attributable risk can estimate the reduction in disease if the factor is removed either in an individual or in a group. This estimate helps to decide about the cost of an intervention or control program versus the benefit of the control of factor or disease in a population.

Examples

Let us hypothetically propose that the incidence rate for oral cancer in young males, ages 25 to 40 years, who use smokeless tobacco for more than 3 years is 24.0 per 1000 and the incidence rate in nonusers is 4.5 per 1000.

1. The relative risk is 24.0/4.5 = 5.3. Those who use smokeless tobacco are over 5 times as likely to get oral cancer than those who do not use smokeless tobacco.

2. The attributable risk for the exposed group, or the excess in incidence rate because of the risk factor, is 24.0 – 4.5 = 19.5.

Thus the excess occurrence of oral cancer among smokeless tobacco users attributed to their use of smokeless tobacco is 19.5 per 1000 users.

3. The attributable risk percentage for the exposed group is 24.0 – 4.5/24.0 = 0.81 or 81%. This would mean that 81% of the oral cancers that occur in young males ages 25 to 40 years who use smokeless tobacco are attributable to that use.

Let's assume that the prevalence of smokeless tobacco use in teenage males is 38% in the general population, then PAR is:

$$0.38 \times (5.3 - 1)/[1 + (0.38 \times (5.3 - 1)] = 0.38 \times 4.3/[1 + (0.38 \times 4.3)] = 1.63/(1 + 1.63) = 0.62.$$

In other words, 62% of oral cancers occurring in all men between the ages of 25 and 40 would be attributable to the use of smokeless tobacco. So, if the use of smokeless tobacco were eliminated, then the excess incidence rate in oral cancer eliminated would be 62 in 1000.

TERMS

Attributable Fraction Population	Same as the attributable fraction exposed except for the entire population
Attributable Proportion	The proportion of the incidence rate that would be reduced from the exposed group if the exposure were eliminated (attributable fraction exposed)
Attributable Risk	The rate of disease in an exposed individual that is due to that exposure
Attributable Risk Percent	The attributable risk expressed as a percent
Population Attributable Risk	The disease incidence in a population that is due to exposure to the factor of interest.

Related Principles
Incidence, prevalence
Relative risk
Odds ratio

References
Cole, P., and MacMahon, B. 1971. Attributable risk percent in case-control studies. Br. J. Prev. Soc. Med. 25:242-244.
Cornfield, J. 1951. A method of estimating comparative rates from clinical data: applications to cancer of the lung, breast, and cervix. J. National Cancer Inst 11:1269-1275.

Kahn, H.A., and Sempos, C.T. 1989. Statistical methods in epidemiology. Monographs in epidemiology and biostatistics, Vol 12. Oxford University Press, New York.

Levin, M.L. 1953. The occurrence of lung cancer in man. Acta Un. Intern. Cancer 19:531-541.

Mausner, J.S., and Kramer, S. 1985. Mausner and Bahn, Epidemiology: an introductory text. W.B. Saunders. Philadelphia, Pennsylvania.

Meittinen, O.S. 1974. Proportion of disease caused or prevented by a given exposure trait or intervention. Am. J. Epidemiol. 99:325-332.

Roht, L.H., Selwyn B.J., Holguin, A.H., and Christensen, B.L. 1982. Principles of epidemiology: a self-teaching guide. Academic Press. Orlando, Florida.

Schlesselman, J.J. 1982. Case-control studies: design, conduct, analysis. Monographs in epidemiology and biostatistics, Vol 2. Oxford University Press, New York.

Walter, S.D. 1976. The estimation and interpretation of attributable risk in health research. Biometrics 32:829-849.

Standardization

Populations that differ significantly in an important host factor or attribute, such as age, which may affect disease, cannot be accurately compared. Instead, the two groups that are to be compared must be "adjusted" or standardized for that factor. Standardization is done by calculating hypothetic rates for each group according to an artificial distribution of that factor that is comparable for both groups.

Explanation

Comparisons between groups yield useful information, but only if the two groups are similar in attributes that may be studied. Unfortunately, in studies that involve observing events as they occur, conditions are not controlled and groups are often dissimilar. Simple summary rates do not reflect group differences that are due to the population's attributes, such as age. The summary rates are an average of the number of individuals and person-time units. Thus comparing summary rates can be misleading. The populations must be adjusted or standardized according to the factor that is different and of interest. Age is a common standardization factor that, when adjusted, results in an age-adjusted rate for both populations. This makes the populations comparable by weighting each population according to the difference in age distribution. Standardization also removes distortion between the populations caused by the differences.

There are two methods of standardization, direct and indirect. Although direct standardization gives a better estimate, the method of standardization depends on what actual information about the population is available. For the direct method of standardization, the attribute-specific rate for each strata within both populations is known. The distribution of the attribute within the populations is not known. Thus the adjustment for the differences between the populations must be done by weighting the attribute's distribution in the two populations with a standard population. For example, the age-specific mortality rate for each age group within the populations may be known but the population distribution is different in each group. The populations must be made more comparable by weighting the factor by a population with a known age distribution. Usually either a commonly available standard population, such as a census population of known age distribution or the larger of the two populations being compared, is chosen as the standard. By applying the age-specific mortality rate in each group to the standard, the result will be the total expected deaths in each group according to a weighted, more similar, distribution. To calculate the age-adjusted mortality rate for each population the new expected deaths are divided by the total standard population.

The indirect method of standardization involves a few more steps than the direct method, but can be calculated with less information about the population under study. The disadvantage of the method is that it is a calculation of a fictional rate and not a true characterization of the population. The specific rate of the attribute of interest, or number of deaths, for each strata within the populations is not known but the distribution of the attribute of interest in the populations is known. The weighting is done by using attribute-specific rates for strata in a standard or known population. The standard population is usually the larger of the two populations because larger populations have stabler rates. Knowing the distribution of the attribute such as age in the population under study and the strata-specific death rate in the standard population allows the calculation of "expected" deaths if the study population were the same as the standard population. It is important that this standard population be reflective of the compared populations so that the "artificial" rates calculated are similar to what the actual rates might be. This makes the fictional rate calculated more representative of the actual rate of the population. For example, the number of individuals in each age group in at least one population should be known. Weighting is done by multiplying the age distribution from the one population with an age-specific mortality rate from the other population or another known population to calculate an age-specific mortality rate for each strata within the populations. The indirect rate is not a characterization of the population but a calculation of some "expected" rate or number. The observed rate is then divided by the expected rate to calculate a

Standardized Mortality Ratio (SMR). If the SMR is larger than 1, it means that more deaths have been observed in the smaller population than would be expected if the smaller population were similar in the attribute of interest to the larger population. Conversely, if the SMR is less than 1, there are fewer deaths observed.

The most important concept to remember is that both methods are simply the process of using a weighting method to make two dissimilar populations with respect to an attribute or factor comparable. But by standardizing the population with an arbitrary standard, the resulting rates are "fictional" and must be interpreted cautiously.

Examples

Death rate resulting from cancer in City X and City Y in 1994. (Fictional data created for this example.)

	CITY X				CITY Y		
Age	Pop.	Deaths	Death Rate		Pop.	Deaths	Death Rate
18-25	5,000	125	0.03		2,000	40	0.02
65-80	800	125	0.16		6,500	800	0.12
Total	5800	250	0.04		8,500	840	0.10

	COMBINED	
Age	Population	Deaths
18-25	7000	165
65-80	7300	925
Total	14,300	1090

Directly comparing the death rates of these two populations would be misleading because the age distributions of the two populations differ greatly. Age does have an effect on the cancer rate because cancer incidence increases with age. The lower cancer death rate in City X may simply be a result of the fact that there are more young individuals in the population and may not be due to the living conditions in City X. To eliminate the effect of age on the outcome of cancer in these two cities, analyses controlling for age need to be done. The crude incidence rates are recalculated as if the two populations had similar age distributions.

1. **Direct method of standardization:**
   a. Merge the two different populations to give a standardized population of two age groups:
   5000 + 2000 (18 to 25 year olds)/14,300 total population, and 800 + 6500 (65 to 80 year olds)/14,300 total population.
   b. Apply the age-specific mortality rates for each city to the standard to calculate age-adjusted mortality rate.

City X
0.03 × 7000 = 210 expected deaths (18 to 25 year olds)
0.16 × 7300 = 1168 expected deaths(65 to 80 year olds)
1378/14,300 = 0.096 (total)

City Y
0.02 × 7000 = 140 expected deaths(18 to 25 year olds)
0.12 × 7300 = 876 expected deaths(65 to 80 year olds)
1016/14300 = 0.071 (total)

The calculated total death rates for City X and City Y are the standardized incidence rates for the two populations. The conclusions are different than without stratification. The ratio of the two standardized incidence rates is 0.096/0.071 = 1.35 and can be used to give an age-standardized comparison of the two populations. In conclusion, individuals in City X are almost 1.4 times more likely to have cancer than in City Y.

2. Indirect method of standardization:
Suppose that the same two cities were to be compared but that certain information about City X was missing. Assume that City X is the exposed population.

	CITY X			**CITY Y**		
Age	**Pop.**	**Deaths**	**Death Rate**	**Pop.**	**Deaths**	**Death Rate**
18-25	5000	?	?	2000	40	0.02
65-80	800	?	?	6500	800	0.12
Total	5800	250		8500	840	0.10

a. The observed number of deaths in the exposed population is 250.
b. The expected number is the number of deaths that would occur if the age-specific death rate were the same in the exposed and reference population.
 Expected death rate in 18 to 25 year olds = 5000 × 0.02 = 100
 Expected death rate in 65 to 80 year olds = 800 × 0.12 = 96
 Total expected deaths would be 196.
c. SMR = observed deaths/expected deaths
 SMR = 250/196 = 1.28
This city has a risk of cancer 28% greater than the reference population or City Y. The SMR indicates an excess risk among those individuals living in City X compared to those individuals in City Y. The magnitude of the excess risk is less than what would be estimated by the relative risk. The SMR always underestimates the true risk.

TERMS

Direct Method	The specific rates for the attribute are known for each strata. A standard population is used to calculate the adjusted specific strata-specific rates
Indirect Method	This method is used when specific rates are unknown. Strata-specific rates from a large or standard population are used to calculate adjusted or standardized rates
Standardization	A statistical method to remove as much as possible the effects of differences in a factor or attribute between two populations when comparing those two populations. This is accomplished by using weighted averaging rates specific for the factor or attribute of interest. The resulting rates are adjusted rates
Standardized Mortality Ratio	Ratio of the number of observed events in the studied population to the number of expected events if the study population had the same specific rates as the standard population

Related Principles
Rates, ratios, proportions
Incidence, prevalence
Person, place, time (Epidemiologic concepts of disease)

References

Kalton, G. 1968. Standardization: a technique to control for extraneous variables. Applied Statistics 17:118-136.

Miettinen, O.S. 1972. Standardization of risk ratios. Am. J. Epidemiol. 96:383-388.

Roht, L.H., Selwyn B.J., Holguin, A.H., and Christensen, B.L. 1982. Principles of epidemiology: a self-teaching guide. Academic Press. Orlando, Florida.

Rothman, K.J. 1986. Modern epidemiology. Little, Brown, and Company. Boston, Massachussetts.

Taylor, J.W. 1977. Simple estimation of population attributable risk for case-control studies. Am. J. Epidemiol. 106: 260.

Walter, S.D. 1975. The distribution of Levin's measure of attributable risk. Biometrika 62: 371-374.

Walter, S.D. 1976. Estimation and interpretation of attributable risk in health research. Biometrics 32: 829-849.

Measures of Frequency and Association: Study Questions

1. Now that you fully understand the method of determining the numerator and denominator, write in formula style and in words the definition for:
   case-fatality rate
   proportional mortality ratio
   age-specific rate
   fertility rate
2. Describe the relevance of using person-time as a denominator in an occupational study of shipbuilders exposed to asbestos or factory workers exposed to a cancer-producing agent.
3. Explain the importance of time in understanding and determining the numerator and denominator, in determining a rate or ratio, and in determining incidence or prevalence.
4. Select 3 or 4 well-known rates and explain why they are or are not ratios.
5. What is the difference between epidemic versus endemic disease? What number of cases determines whether a disease is an epidemic or endemic? Give examples of an epidemic and endemic.
6. What is the difference between incidence and prevalence, and what are the uses of each measure?
7. Explain how a new treatment intervention for a previously fatal acute disease that now creates chronically ill survivors may affect incidence and prevalence rates. Explain what low and high prevalence may signify.
8. Calculate the proper measure of association between age and myocardial infarction for the following information. State why you picked the measure and explain in words what the results show. Would your choice be different if the disease was prostate cancer? Why, or why not?

ACUTE MYOCARDIAL INFARCTION

Age	Yes	No
25-40	125	550
>40	275	345
Total	400	895

9. What is the fundamental difference between a measure of frequency and a measure of association?

10. Explain why the odds ratio is a good approximation of the relative risk when a disease is rare.
11. Explain how you would determine the absolute effect of a factor on the frequency of disease in an individual and in a population. Explain why this information is useful.
12. Why is standardization used? Explain the differences between the direct and indirect method of standardization and when each is used. How do you evaluate the results from each?

CHAPTER 4

Basic Epidemiologic Methodology

Design methodology supplies the tools to question and to study a problem effectively. These tools are basic to any scientific endeavor, whether it is the description of an occurrence of a disease in a population or the determination of the cause of a disease. Once the objective and hypothesis of a study have been decided and the scientific methods of research applied, then the world is yours!

The study **Objective** primarily directs the focus of a descriptive study toward describing the distribution and determinants of a disease in a population and developing a hypothesis. A **Hypothesis** is a conjecture about the cause of disease. Once a hypothesis has been proposed, then rigorous analytic studies are designed to test this conjecture. Depending on the type of study and data collected, different statistical tests and criteria are used to determine if the hypothesis is true.

During the planning stages of a study, criteria must be established so that the results are valid. The **Level of Significance** or alpha level establishes a level or standard on which to decide whether to reject or not to reject the hypothesis. This guideline gives the researcher a certain level of confidence in the conclusions. The probabilities of making a **Type I Error and a Type II Error** are determined before the study to avoid making these errors. A type I or type II error can cause wrong conclusions to be made about the hypothesis.

These same criteria are applied when calculating the **Sample Size** and **Power** needed for the study. Both affect the validity of the study and what conclusions are made about the study. If the sample size is too small, there is a risk of missing important differences in the data and the study may be meaningless. The power of a study is the ability to detect small differences in data. A study loses its usefulness without power.

If the outcome to be evaluated cannot be measured objectively and randomization is not available as a way to prevent bias, then blinding is an alternative. **Blinding** is keeping the subject, observer, or both unaware of the hypothesis or the treatment so that a subjective outcome can be measured as objectively as possible. An example of a subjective outcome measurement would be a certain behavior exhibited or a laboratory test that needs interpretation.

The final step is to determine the type of study that will be conducted, **Experimental** or **Observational.** The main difference is that in the experimental study the researcher has control over the conditions of the experiment and subjects are randomly assigned to the treatment groups. Randomization is the key to making different populations comparable even though they may differ in regards to factors that might be important in the study. Observational methods involve the study of a disease or event as it occurs in the population. Observational studies are common in epidemiology and are covered in depth in Chapter 5. Experimental studies are further differentiated by whether they are **Intervention** or **Therapeutic** trials. The most well-known experimental design is the clinical trial that evaluates the therapeutic value of a treatment in a diseased population. Intervention studies determine the effects of a preventive program on disease in a population. These may be in the form of field trials or large community intervention trials.

List of Principles

Objective and Hypothesis   The starting point of any study design is an objective, hypothesis, or both. An objective usually states a broader goal in order to direct the study. For descriptive studies the objective is to describe the distribution and determinants of disease in the population and to formulate a hypothesis. A hypothesis is an informed guess as to what might be the cause or risk factor of a disease.

Hypothesis Testing   Hypothesis testing allows the epidemiologist to statistically and objectively test a proposed hypothesis. The null hypothesis, which is tested, states that there is no association between two variables, such as exposure and disease. The alternate hypothesis, which is usually what the researcher is interested in, states that there is an association. Because associations cannot really be proven, statistical tests are used to reject or not reject the null hypothesis of no association.

Level of Significance, Type I, Type II Error	The level of significance, type I and type II error are important to establish in the preliminary stages of study design. They are essential in the calculation of sample size and the decision about the hypothesis testing at the end of the study.
Sample Size	Sample size must be large enough at the beginning of study to have enough statistical power to detect the differences deemed important. Sample size calculations are based on a number of factors within the study design such as prevalence, acceptable error, and the detectable difference.
Blinding	Blinding is used to keep potentially subjective outcomes measured as objectively as possible. Blinding involves keeping the subject, researcher, or both unaware of the treatment or the study hypothesis.
Experimental versus Observational	The fundamental difference between experimental and observational studies is that in an experimental study the researcher controls the conditions of the experiment. Randomization is often an important factor in the control. Observational studies have no intervention by the researcher and are observations and analyses of the event as it happens or after it has happened.
Therapeutic versus Intervention	Experimental studies can be further delineated by whether they involve looking at the therapeutic value of a treatment or looking at the results of a prevention program on disease. Clinical trials are the most common experimental studies designed to evaluate therapies. Field and community trials evaluate the effect of prevention strategies on the occurrence of disease.

Objective and Hypothesis

The starting point of any study design is an objective, hypothesis, or both. An objective usually states a broader goal in order to direct the study. For descriptive studies the objective is to describe the distribution and determinants of disease in the population and to formulate a hypothesis. A hypothesis is an informed guess as to what might be the cause or risk factor of a disease.

Explanation

The basic starting point of any study or experiment is an objective and a hypothesis. These two terms may be used similarly but denote different meanings. An objective clarifies the purpose or the goal of the study. It is the initial point for designing and directing the type of study needed to achieve the objective. There may be several objectives, especially if the goal is to explore or describe the distribution of the disease in the population or to look for possible risk factors for the disease. The objective is often linked to a descriptive type of study that characterizes the distribution of disease in the population and trends in person, place, and time. Although there may be several objectives, it is important to keep the objectives as clear and as focused as possible to obtain useful data. Too many objectives will collect voluminous data that are both confusing and useless. An important goal for a descriptive study is to collect enough right information to formulate a hypothesis about the association of risk factors for a disease.

A hypothesis is an informed guess or conjecture about the association of two or more variables that can be tested by a study. The variables of interest are risk factors that may be associated with disease. Ultimately, epidemiologists are searching for the actual causes of disease. The hypothesis implies that all the variables, both the risk factors and the disease, can be measured and also specifies how they are to be measured. Like an objective, the hypothesis directs the epidemiologist as to the type of study needed to test this hypothesis. It is important to test only one or two hypotheses, although there is a tendency to look at several. Multiple testing of hypotheses can increase the likelihood for significant results to be lost.

Example

There has been one report in the literature about an ACE (acteylcholinesterase) inhibitor used for blood pressure causing an anaphylactoid reaction in certain dialysis patients right after they start dialysis. An anaphylactoid reaction is one that resembles anaphylaxis. Anaphylaxis is an allergic reaction that is exaggerated or unusual; it can be fatal.

An objective for a descriptive study might be stated as:

This preliminary study will look at a population of dialysis patients to determine if those patients on angiotension-converting enzyme (ACE) inhibitors have more anaphylactoid reactions on certain dialysis systems.

After a descriptive study is done, it has been determined that certain types of dialyzers seem to cause more reactions in dialysis patients who are on ACE inhibitors. A hypothesis for an analytic study to be tested might be stated as:

> The use of ACE inhibitors within 24 hours of dialysis treatment and the concomitant use of a polyacrylonitrile dialyzer membrane increases the risk of the patient having an anaphylactoid reaction.

TERMS

Hypothesis   An informed guess or conjecture as to the association of two variables or the cause of a disease

Objective   The clear, focused purpose or goal of a study

Related Principles
Person, place, and time (Epidemiologic concepts of disease)
Hypothesis testing
Cross-sectional, survey studies (Observational studies)
Experimental, observational studies
Therapeutic versus intervention
Critical reasoning (Overview)
Natural, ecologic studies (Observational studies)

References

Hennekens, C.H., Buring, J.E., and edited by S.L. Mayrent. 1987. Epidemiology in medicine. Little, Brown, and Company. Boston, Massachusetts.
Kerlinger, F.N. 1986. Foundations of behavioral research. Third edition. CBS College Publishing, Holt, Rinehart, and Winston. New York.

Hypothesis Testing

Hypothesis testing allows the epidemiologist to statistically and objectively test a proposed hypothesis. The null hypothesis, which is tested, states that there is no association between two variables, such as exposure and disease. The alternate hypothesis, which is usually what the researcher is interested in, states there is an association. Because associations cannot really be proven, statistical tests are used to reject or not reject the null hypothesis of no association.

Explanation

Once an informed guess has been made about the cause of the disease, there must be a method to find out if the guess is correct. The study hypothesis is tested by a scientific study and an analysis of the results. In statistical terms, the hypothesis to be tested is considered to be the null hypothesis that can be stated either in words or as a formula. The null hypothesis states that there is no association or no true difference between the groups to be compared with respect to the variable of interest. For instance, there is no difference in the disease rate between a treated group and a nontreated group. The null hypothesis is saying that the results of the study could have occurred simply as a result of chance and are not because of the true differences between the groups. If this is true, then the informed guess about the cause of a disease is incorrect. The null hypothesis states that there is no association because statistically an association cannot be proven, only estimated.

The alternate hypothesis is really the informed guess that the epidemiologists have formed about the cause or risk factors of a disease. If the null hypothesis is rejected, then the alternate hypothesis is correct. The alternate hypothesis states that there is a difference between the groups or an association between the variables. The association between variables could be positive or negative. For example, an exposure to a particular factor could cause an increased risk of disease, or an exposure to a factor could cause a decreased risk in disease. Sometimes it is unclear in what direction the association may be. Thus the alternate hypothesis is broadly worded so that the results have a better chance of fitting under the alternate hypothesis. The alternate hypothesis may be considered statistically as one-sided or two-sided; this decision influences the type of statistical level used in testing the hypothesis. One-sided means the direction of the difference is known. For instance, the untreated group will have more disease than the treated group, or a group exposed to a particular variable is more diseased than a group not exposed. Two-sided is commonly used because the direction of effect is often unknown. It states no direction, only that there is a difference.

Once a hypothesis is formulated, then an analytic study is designed to test the hypothesis. Depending on the type of study and data collected, there are various statistical tests used to determine if the null hypothesis of no association is true. A significant statistical test shows that there is a difference between the groups and that the null hypothesis should be rejected. The test to determine statistical significance is determined by the type of data collected in the study. For example, continuous data, such as number counts, require one type of statistical test and categoric data, such as a yes or no answer, require another type of statistical test. A large statistical test value usually means there is a true significant statistical difference between the groups and that the result was not due to chance or error.

The two main criteria used in conjunction with the statistical test to determine if a result is truly statistically significant are the p-value (probability) and the confidence interval. Statistical tests, such as a chi-square test, calculate a p-value or a probability statement. The larger the statistical test value, the lower the p-value. In fact, the use of p-values is often called significance testing. The p-value assumes the null hypothesis is true and represents the probability that an association of the same magnitude seen in the study data might have been caused by chance or by some random error. A low p-value means that the probability is low that the null hypothesis is true and that the data are more compatible with the alternate hypothesis. The null hypothesis is rejected, and the difference is considered statistically significant. If the p-value is <0.05, then there is less than a 5 in a 100 chance of the results seen in the study occurring by chance. The association is considered statistically significant if the p-value of 0.05 is selected as the value cut-off for statistical significance at the beginning of the study. It is important to realize that the p-value is *not* the probability that the null hypothesis is true.

One disadvantage of the p-value is that it is affected by variation between groups and sample size. Consequently, small differences might be considered statistically significant if the sample size is large enough, and an important effect might not be statistically significant if the sample size is too small. The confidence interval supplies extra information that the p-value does not; it evaluates the variability of the estimated observed values for the study and the magnitude of the association. Therefore the confidence interval also needs to be considered with the p-value in deciding whether to reject or not to reject the null hypothesis.

The confidence interval calculates a range of possible estimates within which the observed values could fall. The width of the range depends on the variability in the data and the level of confidence or consistency of the data. The sample size influences the variability of the data. The larger the sample size, the less the variability in the data. A large sample size ensures that all of the variability or differences among individuals "evens out." A wide confidence interval denotes a large amount of variation and possible error. The narrower the confidence interval, the less the variability. If the confidence interval contains one, the results are considered not significant.

The decision about whether the hypothesis is correct or not is guided by the statistical significance of the tests and the criteria set for the hypothesis testing. Both the p-value (probability) and the confidence interval are needed to make the decision. Finally, the results must also make biologic and plausible sense. The testing may be statistically significant but not have a plausible, biologic explanation. Likewise, something might not be statistically significant, but it may have an effect biologically.

Examples

1. There is an interest in whether people with asthma are more likely to have asthma attacks if they own pets. Therefore the null hypothesis is that asthmatic patients are no more likely to have asthma attacks if they own a pet than those asthmatics who do not have pets. Of course, the alternate hypothesis is that asthmatic individuals who own pets are more likely to have asthma attacks than asthmatics who do not have pets. A sample of asthmatic patients is taken from family practitioners' medical records to see if those patients reporting asthmatic attacks own pets.

DISEASE (Asthma attack in the last 24 hours)

Exposure (Pets)	Yes	No	Total
Yes	33	45	78
No	30	45	75
Total	63	90	153

Incidence rate (IR) of asthma attacks with pets equals 33/78.
Incidence rate of asthma attacks without pets equals 30/75.
Relative risk (RR) equals IR with pets/IR without pets.
Relative risk equals 33/78/30/75 = 1.06.
Chi-Square test values equals 0.08 with a p-value of 0.77.
Confidence interval equals 0.72 < RR < 1.55.

The p-value is greater than 0.05 and the confidence interval, though narrow, includes 1 so the statistical test is not significant. Therefore the null hypothesis is not rejected and the conclusion is that pet ownership is not a risk for asthma attacks.

2. Suppose that the incidence rates were different and that the calculated relative risk = 1.7. The chi-square value was 4.63 with a p-value of 0.03 and a confidence interval of 0.98 < RR < 15.85. What would you conclude?

    Although the p-value is 0.03 and less than 0.05 and the RR = 1.7 and it looks like there is a risk, the confidence interval is broad and includes 1. The value is still not considered statistically significant and the null hypothesis should not be rejected.

3. You are still not convinced that pets are not a risk factor for asthma attacks, so a larger sample of patients is taken from several geographic regions.

DISEASE

Exposure	Yes	No	Total
Yes	200	10	210
No	300	150	450
Total	500	160	660

The incidence rate of disease with a pet equals 200/210.
The incidence rate of disease without a pet equals 300/450.
Relative risk equals 1.43.
Chi-Square test value equals 63.64 with a p-value of 0.0000.
Confidence interval equals $1.33 < RR < 1.54$.

These results show a statistically significant result. Therefore reject the null hypothesis and conclude that the alternate hypothesis is true.

TERMS

Alternate Hypothesis	Is usually the hypothesis of the informed guess and states that there is a difference between the variables studied
Confidence Interval	Range of values that have a probability that the range will contain the true value of interest. End points of the range are the confidence limits
Null Hypothesis	States that there is no difference between treatments or populations or no association between exposure and disease. The testing of this hypothesis will result in a decision to either reject or not to reject the hypothesis
One-Sided	The direction of the effect of the variable is known and stated
P-Value	The probability that data of the same magnitude as the study results may have occurred by chance assuming there is really no difference between the groups (null hypothesis)
Statistical Significance	Determined by statistical tests, the p-value, and confidence interval. A conclusion that the study results are not due to chance

Two-Sided The direction of effect of the variable is unknown so the hypothesis is stated more broadly. It merely states that there is a difference

---

Related Principles
Objective and hypothesis
Sample size
Level of significance, type I and type II error

References
Huck, S.W., Cormier, W.H., Bounds, W.G. 1974. Reading statistics and research. Harper and Row, New York.

Ott, L. 1984. An introduction to statistical methods and data analysis. Second edition. PWS Publishers. Boston, Massachusetts.

Rothman, K.J. 1986. Modern epidemiology. Little, Brown, and Company. Boston, Massachusetts.

Zar, J.H. 1984. Biostatistical analysis. Second edition. Prentice Hall. Englewood Cliffs, New Jersey.

Level of Significance, Type I and Type II Error

The level of significance, type I and type II error are important to establish in the preliminary stages of study design. They are essential in the calculation of sample size and the decision about the hypothesis testing at the end of the study.

Explanation

Several criteria have to be determined in the designing of a study; one of these is the level of significance or alpha (α). The level of significance, or alpha, is the chance a researcher is willing to take in incorrectly rejecting the null hypothesis. The level chosen at the beginning of the study planning is arbitrary but the two most common values are 0.01 and 0.05. The "stricter" level is 0.01. A level of significance of 0.01 means that in repeating the study 100 times only one of those replications might give the same results as the observed values by chance. Then, if the results are significant, the difference is true and not due to chance. It also makes sense that the tougher the criteria, the more confidence there is in the results and conclusions. Indeed, the level of confidence is related to the level of significance; $1 - \alpha =$ level of confidence. A level of significance of 0.01 has a 0.99 level of confidence. The results of the study will be the same as the observed in 99 out of 100 replications of the study.

The level of significance, or alpha, is the probability of making the type I error. Type I error is the mistake of rejecting the null hypothesis when it is actually true. If the level of significance is 0.01, then there is a probability of 0.01 or (1 out of 100) that the null hypothesis will be rejected when it is actually true. In other words, a statistical difference is demonstrated when there is none. It makes sense that to prevent a type I error the alpha level must be set at low values, such as 0.01 or 0.001.

The probabilities of both type I and type II error need to be determined in the preliminary stages of designing a study. Type I and type II error criteria help to prevent these errors, to calculate sample size, and to make a decision about the hypothesis testing. Type II error is accepting the null hypothesis when it should be rejected or simply missing a difference that exists between the groups being compared. Beta (β) is the probability of committing the type II error. Type II error is also related to power in that $1 - \beta$ = power. Power is the ability to accurately pick up and estimate a difference in groups or an effect, or the probability of rejecting the hypothesis when it is actually false. Depending on how much of a difference needs to be detected determines the value of β that is selected.

In setting the alpha and beta levels in the preliminary stages of design, both cannot be minimized at the same time. Logically, it is not possible to prevent the rejection of the null hypothesis when it is true or to prevent the acceptance of the null hypothesis when it is false at the same time. As alpha decreases, beta increases. A lower alpha value that is established as the cut off for statistical significance means that there is a greater chance to commit a type II error when there is an effect. A decision must be made as to what is the most important standard.

Examples
1. Typical 2 × 2 table and the probability of committing a type I and type II error.

DISEASE

Risk Factor	Yes	No
Yes		type II error
No	type I error	

2. Example of how the sample size varies with the predetermined values of alpha and beta and a constant risk or difference to be detected. Assume risk to be detected is 1.5. Assume the proportion of the control group exposed is 10%.

ALPHA	BETA	SAMPLE SIZE
0.01	0.01	2795
0.01	0.05	2065
0.01	0.10	1728
0.01	0.20	1357
0.05	0.10	1217
0.05	0.20	910
0.10	0.10	989
0.10	0.20	713

Schlesselman, J.J. 1982. Case-control studies: design, conduct, analysis. Monographs in epidemiology and biostatistics, Vol 2. Oxford University Press, New York.

3. The effect of the alpha, beta level, and sample size, on the detection of a difference or relative risk. The table demonstrates the largest and smallest detectable relative risk. Assume the proportion of the control group exposed is 50%.

		BETA					
	sample	0.01		0.05		0.10	
alpha	size	max.	min.	max.	min.	max.	min.
0.01	25	>50	0.02	15.6	0.1	10.6	0.1
	50	8.0	0.1	5.5	0.2	4.6	0.2
	200	2.6	0.4	2.2	0.5	2.1	0.5
0.05	25	15.6	0.1	8.0	0.1	6.0	0.2
	50	5.5	0.2	4.0	0.3	3.4	0.3
	200	2.2	0.5	1.9	0.5	1.8	0.6

Max., Maximum detectable relative risk; *min.*, minimum detectable relative risk. Schlesselman, J.J. 1982. Case-control studies: design, conduct, analysis. Monographs in epidemiology and biostatistics, Vol. 2. Oxford University Press, New York.

TERMS

Alpha	The probability of committing the type I error, also the level of significance
Beta	The probability of committing the type II error
Level of Significance	A value that sets an acceptable magnitude of type I error

Power   The ability to accurately determine a difference between the means

Type I Error   The error of rejecting the null hypothesis when it is actually not true. The error of seeing a difference when there is none

Type II Error   The error of not rejecting the null hypothesis when it is actually false. The error of missing a difference between the means

Related Principles
Sample size
Hypothesis testing

References
Freiman, J., Chalmers, T.C., Smith, H., and Kuebler, R.R. 1978. The importance of beta, the type II error and sample size in the design and interpretation of the randomized control trial. New Engl. J. Med. 299:690-694.

Hennekens, C.H., Buring, J.E., and S.L. Mayrent (ed). 1987. Epidemiology in medicine. Little, Brown, and Company. Boston, Massachusetts.

Rothman, K.J. 1986. Modern epidemiology. Little, Brown, and Company. Boston, Massachusetts.

Schlesselman, J.J. 1982. Case-control studies: design, conduct, analysis. Monographs in epidemiology and biostatistics, Vol 2. Oxford University Press, New York.

Sample Size

Sample size must be large enough at the beginning of study to have enough statistical power to detect the differences deemed important. Sample size calculations are based on a number of factors within the study design such as prevalence, acceptable error, and the detectable difference.

Explanation

The time and expense of studies warrant that they be done correctly so that results are valid and the data obtained are useful. Sample size is an important consideration for the design of any study. The sample size must be large enough to detect important differences between groups being studied or to detect significant associations between an exposure and a disease. If the sample size is too small, only a very large difference will be detected between the groups. Important smaller differences that may give a clue to a risk factor for a disease might be missed. This would be a type II error. It is important for epidemiologists to determine before the study how big or how small a difference they want to detect between groups.

There are various factors that affect the sample size and, therefore, are included in most of the formulas used to calculate the sample size. Because the sample size has to be large enough to detect a difference, an estimate is needed of how much of a difference or delta (d), that needs to be detected. A larger difference is easier to detect and requires a smaller sample size. The frequency or prevalence of the disease in the groups is also a factor. The more common the disease, the smaller sample size is needed. As mentioned previously, sample size calculation also depends on type I and type II error, and power. If the study is one that follows subjects over time, the sample size also needs to be enlarged to take into consideration that some subjects will drop out. The sample size that is determined is the number of the sample that is required at the end of the study after the loss of subjects over time.

In the beginning of designing a study, it is a good idea to organize a table of sample sizes calculated according to different prevalences, power, acceptable error, and significance levels so that a determination of the best possible sample size can be made. Sample size formulas depend on the hypothesis, the type of study, and the data to be collected. Various formulas can be found in textbooks and even in computer statistical packages. There are many circumstances where there are limitations of cost, time, and rarity of the disease. In that case, the most important factor is that the study have enough power for the results to be valid. Power can be increased only by increasing the precision of measurement, increasing the sample size, or decreasing the type II error.

Example

A study is planned to look at an exposed group with a 10% prevalence of disease. Alpha is set at 0.05. You want to calculate the power and sample size needed to detect a 10% change in the prevalence.

POWER	SAMPLE SIZE
90%	240
80%	190
70%	158
50%	112

These calculations change depending on the prevalence of the disease or factor in the population. For example, if the prevalence of disease in the exposed population is 50%, then for 80% power a sample size of 28 is needed. At the same time, if the disease in the exposed is only 1%, a sample size of 2542 is needed. Therefore the lower the prevalence of disease, the larger the sample size.

TERMS

Power	The ability to accurately determine a difference between the means $(1 - \beta)$ (probability of committing type II error)
Sample Size	The number of individuals needed in a study to achieve the objective or prove the hypothesis

Related Principles
Level of significance, type I and type II error
Hypothesis testing

Classic citation
Fleiss, J.L. 1981. Statistical methods for rates and proportions, Second edition. John Wiley and Sons, New York.

References
Meinert, C.L. 1986. Clinical trials: design, conduct, analysis. Monographs in epidemiology and biostatistics. Vol 8. Oxford University Press, New York.
Rothman, K.J. 1986. Modern epidemiology. Little, Brown, and Company. Boston, Massachusetts.
Schlesselman, J.J. 1982. Case-control studies: design, conduct, analysis. Monographs in epidemiology and biostatistics, Vol 2. Oxford University Press, New York.

Blinding

Blinding is used to keep potentially subjective outcomes measured as objectively as possible. Blinding involves keeping the subject, researcher, or both unaware of the treatment or the study hypothesis.

Explanation

Blinding, or masking, helps prevent partial observations and results, particularly when the outcome being measured is subjective. Blinding can be accomplished in two ways. Blinding can be done by keeping study subjects involved in clinical trials unaware of the type of treatment they are receiving. This keeps the subject behavior as objective as possible. This does not mean that research subjects are unaware of being studied; there must be informed consent. They are just unaware as to what effect the researcher thinks the treatment will have. Single-blinded means that only the subject is blinded to the treatment or hypothesis.

Blinding can also be accomplished by keeping the observers or interpreters of the outcome unaware of the hypothesis or treatment. This is especially important if the outcome measurement could be subjective. Blinding keeps the measurements as objective as possible. Double-blinded studies are studies in which the subject and the observer are unaware of the treatment or hypothesis. Triple-blinding is rare and involves even the data analyzer being unaware of the hypothesis.

Blinding is useful in experimental studies in which the subject's knowledge about a new drug might affect the response to questions about physical or mental condition. If the subject believes the new drug will work, then the subject may report feeling better even if the drug is not effective. In this case, the ineffective drug may be acting as a placebo. A related phenomenon is the placebo effect. This occurs when an individual reports an effect of the treatment even when receiving an inert medication or placebo. When subjects are assigned to different treatment groups, neither the observer nor the subject should know which treatment they are receiving. In this way, all groups will be treated equally. If these conditions are met, then the effect observed can be attributed only to the real effect of the treatments and not to subjective evaluations or feelings.

Blinding is important in observational studies especially in surveys involving face-to-face interviews. If the interviewer is not blinded, they could influence the subject by nonverbal or even verbal cues to get the desired response. Observers measuring subjective outcomes, such as behavior or the interpretation of laboratory tests, who are unaware of the hypothesis are more likely to report unbiased results rather than report results that might prove a hypothesis.

Examples

1. Two different drugs and a placebo are being compared in clinical trials for the treatment of postpartum depression in women. One drug is already approved for treatment for depression and the other drug is being tested for its effectiveness. Data collection involves a questionnaire filled out by the women about how they feel and a questionnaire filled out by family members about the behavior of the women. Blinding to the treatment and to the hypothesis for the subjects and their families is essential to see if the drugs really work. If women and/or the families are aware of the treatment, then their responses to the questionnaires may be influenced by what treatment group they are in.
2. An observational study involves asking a group of individuals diagnosed with malignant melanoma, and a comparable group of individuals without malignant melanoma, about past sun exposure and

severe sunburns. If the individuals are aware that severe sunburns caused by an acute exposure to sun are linked to malignant melanoma, they are more likely, especially the diseased individuals, to recall any type of sun exposure. Recall of events is usually more complete when it involves a serious or life-threatening event or illness.

TERMS

Blinded Study	A study when the subject, researcher, or both are unaware of the treatment or the hypothesis
Double-Blinded	The subject and observer are unaware of the treatment or hypothesis
Placebo	An inert medication
Placebo Effect	A subject reports a physiologic effect of the medication even though it is inert
Single-Blinded	The subject is unaware of the treatment or hypothesis
Triple-Blinded	Subject, observer, and even the data analyzer are unaware of the hypothesis

Related Principles
Selection bias (Bias and error)
Information bias (Bias and error)
Experimental versus observational
Cross-sectional, survey studies (Observational studies)

References
Hennekens, C.H., Buring, J.E., and edited by S.L. Mayrent. 1987. Epidemiology in medicine. Little, Brown, and Company. Boston, Massachusetts.

Lilienfeld, A.M., Lilienfeld, D.E. 1980. Foundations of epidemiology. Second edition. Oxford University Press, New York. Revised by Lilienfeld, D.E., Stolley, P.D. (eds.) 1994. Foundation of epidemiology, Third edition. Oxford University Press, New York.

Experimental versus Observational

The fundamental difference between experimental and observational studies is that in an experimental study the researcher controls the conditions of the experiment. Randomization is often an important factor in the control. Observational studies have no intervention by the researcher and are observations and analyses of the event as it happens or after it has happened.

Explanation

Experimental and observational studies have different goals in the study of disease. Clinical researchers are interested in the treatment of disease, whereas epidemiologists are interested in finding the cause and prevention of a disease. With experimental design, the researcher controls all of the conditions of the experiment. One of the main components of the control is the randomization of individuals into the different treatment or exposure groups of interest. Randomization allows the comparability among the groups and "evens out" possible differences in the groups that are unknown. It gives each individual an opportunity to be treated or exposed and to be affected by that treatment or exposure. Ideally then, the results of the study can be attributed entirely to the treatment or exposure being studied and not to unrelated differences among the groups. One variable at a time can be studied. Through replications of the experiment, different variables of interest can be manipulated one at a time to determine their effect. This is advantageous since most outcomes are influenced by several factors that are hard to delineate. The experimental design is thought to be the paradigm of scientific research.

Unfortunately, many diseases cannot be studied in an experimental setting. The study of exposures to environmental toxins or the dietary habits of diabetics cannot be done under controlled situations. Ethically, experimental trials may not be done because of the seriousness of the disease and the impropriety of keeping a new treatment from seriously ill individuals. Time and cost also limit the use of experimental studies. The observational design is an alternative in which to study diseases or exposures in the populations in which they are occurring.

Observational studies evaluate the effect of an exposure that has already happened or attempt to determine the cause of a disease or an event that has already occurred. To do this, the study requires a group that has been exposed or has the disease or event of interest and a comparable group without the exposure or disease. There are different names for each group depending on the type of observational study selected (Chapter 5). Both groups need to be representative of the general population that is exposed or diseased, and the groups need to be similar to each other in every aspect except the variable being studied. Other differences between the groups could affect the results of the study.

Observational studies are advantageous in that they are easier to complete, more rapid, and less expensive. Because the epidemiologist has less control over the conditions of the study, there is some lack of trust among the scientific community in the results for observational studies. There is more concern about the results being a result of other factors not controlled rather than the variable of interest. Careful study design and selection of representative groups can make these studies as valuable as randomized clinical trials. Because randomization is not possible in observational studies, other strategies are used to simulate the effects of randomization and to make the groups comparable except for the variable being studied.

Examples

Consider studying the effect of cholesterol levels on coronary heart disease.

1. **Experimental:** Individuals have volunteered for a study on the effects of diet on cholesterol and the consequential effect of cholesterol on the incidence of coronary heart disease. These individuals are randomly assigned to three types of diets with varying levels of fat, protein, and carbohydrates. The subjects have agreed to adhere to the assigned diet for a period of one year. Cholesterol levels and medical history are taken before and after the change in diet.

2. **Observational:** a. A long-term study is planned to determine the effects of cholesterol and diet on myocardial infarction. A population (e.g., Framingham or Nurse's Health Study) is selected to participate in the study. This large group of individuals agree to fill out a questionnaire about their exercise patterns, smoking history, family history, medical history, and current medications. They also agree to keep a diary of the food they eat weekly for one year. At the end of the year, a physical exam and a medical chart review are done to evaluate coronary heart status. The food entries from the diaries are categorized into approximate levels of fat, protein, and carbohydrates.

b. Another option would be evaluate two groups of patients from participating hospitals. One group was hospitalized because of coronary heart disease, and the other group was hospitalized for other reasons. The medical records for both groups are abstracted for the past year to see if cholesterol levels are available. In addition, patients are administered a questionnaire to ask about diet in the last year, medical and family history, and current medications. The cholesterol levels and diet in the coronary diseased group can be compared to the group without coronary disease to see if the cholesterol levels and diet have an effect.

TERMS

Experimental	A study where all conditions are controlled by the researcher and subjects are often randomized to different treatment groups
Observational	A study that observes the differences in groups of the factor of question and analyzes those differences without intervention or control by the researcher
Randomization	Selection or allocation of subjects into groups by chance, and each individual has the same opportunity of being in the group

Related Principles
Therapeutic versus intervention
Blinding
Case-control, retrospective studies (Observational studies)
Prospective, cohort studies (Observational studies)
Cross-sectional, survey studies (Observational studies)

References
Kelsey, J.L., Thompson, W.D., Evans, A.S. 1986. Methods in observational epidemiology. Monographs in epidemiology and biostatistics. Vol 10. Oxford University Press, New York.
Meinert, C.L. 1986. Clinical trials: design, conduct, analysis. Monographs in epidemiology and biostatistics. Vol 8. Oxford University Press, New York.

Therapeutic versus Intervention

Experimental studies can be further delineated by whether they involve looking at the therapeutic value of a treatment or the results of a prevention program on disease. Clinical trials are the most common experimental studies designed to evaluate therapies. Field and community trials evaluate the effect of prevention strategies on the occurrence of disease.

Explanation

Controlled, randomized clinical trials are considered the "gold standard" of experimental design. Although observational studies are more common in epidemiology, clinical trials are used. Most often clinical trials are used to evaluate the therapeutic value of a treatment in a population of individuals. The subjects are randomly assigned to one or more groups. One or more groups receive the treatments of interest and one group, referred to as the control, receives a placebo or no treatment. There are some instances where there is a placebo group and a no-treatment group. It is important for the validity of the study to ensure that even though the control group is not receiving a treatment they are otherwise treated exactly the same way as the experimental groups so that the only difference is the treatment.

Unlike clinical trials, field and community trials often involve studying the effect of preventive programs or a particular intervention in a healthy population. Prevention means prohibiting a disease from occurring; intervention can be a form of prevention. Intervention is an action that changes the effect of a risk factor or the progress of a disease. Both field and community trials involve determining the efficacy of preventive programs such as vaccination, screening, or intervention in a population. Field trials, although done in large populations, still look at the effect of the intervention on the individual within that entire population. Depending on the incidence of the disease in the population, a large sample size is needed for field trials. The actual number of healthy individuals that become ill is small. Most field trials are limited to very serious, or very common diseases, or to individuals at very high risk because of the large number of individuals required and the cost. Field trials also cover a large geographic area, which adds expense and complexity.

A larger expansion of the field trial is a community intervention trial that studies the effects of an intervention on an entire community or population. Unlike the field trial where the prevention focuses on the individual, these preventive interventions can only be implemented on the community as a whole. Community trials can be done in military units, universities, or whole communities.

Examples

1. Clinical trials:

A randomized clinical trial to test whether aspirin, ibuprofen, or acetaminophen is most effective in relief of pain in arthritic patients.

A population of arthritic patients is recruited. Patients are randomly assigned to four different groups: a group being treated with aspirin, a group being treated with ibuprofen, a group being treated with acetaminophen, and a group being treated with a placebo. Treatment is prescribed for two months. At that time, a questionnaire is filled out by the patients about the amount of pain they experienced, mobility, and their quality of life. Blinding would be important in this trial.

2. **Field trials:**
   a. Trials of an oral vaccine against rabies in wildlife have been used in Europe since the 1980s to decrease the incidence and spread of fox rabies. The rabies vaccine is a recombinant vaccine that is placed in bait that the wildlife ingests. The baits are dropped by airplane or by hand in selected geographic areas. Field trials for oral vaccination of raccoons have been conducted in the eastern states to prevent the further spread of raccoon rabies and to prevent further transmission of the disease from wildlife to domestic animals.
   b. Salk's polio vaccination trials. Polio caused death and permanent disability in children in the 1940s and 1950s. Jonas Salk developed a vaccine that he felt would protect children against polio and prevent further disease. Early in the 1950s almost a million children were randomized into two groups, one receiving Salk's experimental vaccine and the other receiving a placebo. This large trial proved the safety and effectiveness of the vaccine.

3. **Community trials:**
   Fluoridation of drinking water to prevent dental caries. This was carried out by the United States Public Health Service in the 1940s to see if fluoride added to drinking water would decrease the risk of dental caries in children. The Newburgh, New York community had fluoride added to their water supply while the water supply in Kingston, New York remained unfluoridated. The results showed a significant reduction over time in dental caries in Newburgh.

TERMS

Clinical Trial	A research study that determines the efficacy and safety of a drug or treatment method in subjects that are randomized
Community Trial	Usually a larger extension of a field trial that studies the effects of an intervention on an entire community
Field Trial	A research study that evaluates the effect of an intervention on disease occurrence at an individual level within an entire population

Related Principles
Blinding
Experimental versus observational
Prevention and control (Overview)

Classic Citations

Ast, D.B., Finn, S.B., and McCaffrey, I. 1950. The Newburgh-Kingston caries fluorine study: I. Dental findings after three years of water fluoridation. Am. J. Public Health 40: 716-724.

Ast, D.B., and Schlesinger, E.R. 1956. The conclusion of a ten-year study of water fluoridation. Am. J. Public Health. 46:265-271.

Francis, T.F, Korns, R.F., Voight, R.B. et al. 1955. An evaluation of the 1954 poliomyelitis vaccine trials. Am. J. of Public Health 45 (May supplement): 1-63.

References

Brochier, B., Kieny, M.P., Costy, F. et al. 1991. Large scale eradication of rabies using recombinant vaccinia-rabies vaccine. Nature 354: 520-522.

Meinert, C.L. 1986. Clinical trials: design, conduct, analysis. Monographs in epidemiology and biostatistics, Vol 8. Oxford University Press, New York.

Basic Epidemiologic Methodology: Study Questions

1. There has been an outbreak of pyrogenic reactions in one dialysis center in the last week. A pyrogenic reaction is a fever produced by an endotoxin. It may be related to the water treatment systems in the dialysis facility that takes the community water supply, treats the water, and then uses it in the dialysis process.
   State a study objective that might be proposed.
      There are reports that the water treatment systems do not always contain all of the necessary components, such as filters, to purify the water. Also, there are times when the water treatment systems do not function properly.
   Think about a possible hypothesis for this problem and state it. How would you design this study?
2. Why is there a null hypothesis and an alternate hypothesis? Explain the differences between the two and the significance of the two in hypothesis testing. When is the two-sided statistical test more appropriate?
3. Explain in words what a p-value of 0.01 means.
4. Should the p-value or the confidence interval be used in the decision of whether the result is statistically significant? Explain your answer.

5. What influence does sample size have on the p-value and the confidence interval?
6. Explain the relationships of α and β, type I and type II error, sample size, and power.
7. What is the importance of sample size to the proper design of a study?
8. Give examples of field and community trials not mentioned in this chapter.
9. Explain the main differences between an experimental and an observational study. Give a situation that needs to be studied experimentally, and then describe a situation that can only be studied by an observational design.
10. Describe a study that needs to be blinded to achieve valid results. Describe a study requiring single-blinding and one requiring double-blinding.
11. You have conducted a clinical trial to determine the effectiveness of either Tagamet, Zantac, and each drug together with antacids in preventing the recurrence of duodenal ulcers in patients previously diagnosed with ulcers. At the end of a six month treatment, the number of recurring ulcers is measured and each patient fills out a questionnaire about painful symptoms. You get a hypothesis test value of 54.19 with a p-value of 0.02. You also calculate a confidence interval of 32.16 to 58.44. What are your conclusions? Would your conclusions be the same if you had a confidence interval of 2.19 to 126.77? What if you got a test value of 4.77 and a p-value of 0.86? State what all of your conclusions are in words and whether you reject or do not reject the null hypothesis.
12. You have been asked to design a study. You will have limited resources and therefore a limited sample size. The level of significance is fixed at 0.10, and you must decide between the probability of committing a type I error (rejecting a true null hypothesis) or the probability of committing a type II error (accepting a false null hypothesis). Describe a study question where it would be more important to prevent a type I error and then describe a study question where it would be more important to prevent a type II error. What would changing the level of significance to 0.01 do?

CHAPTER 5

Observational Studies

Observational studies evaluate the effect of an exposure that has already occurred or determine a cause of a disease or event that has already happened. To do this, the study compares two groups, one that has been exposed or has the disease of interest, and a similar group without the exposure or disease. Observational studies include those designed to provide descriptive information about the distribution of the disease in a population, to provide possible risk factors, and to formulate hypotheses about the disease and its risk factors. They also include analytic studies designed to test proposed hypotheses and to determine associations between risk factors and a disease. The eventual goal of any epidemiologic study is to determine the cause of disease and the effect of a control measure on that disease. It is important to realize that in designing observational studies the same methodological issues addressed in Chapter 4, such as sample size, power, and level of significance, must be considered (Fig. 5-1).

Each type of descriptive study has advantages and disadvantages. A **Natural Experiment** is a rare occurrence but offers a unique opportunity to observe and gain information about an exposure that occurs in a natural setting. For example, the unfortunate nuclear radiation leak at Three Mile Island, Pennsylvania, enabled epidemiologists to observe the effects of radiation on humans, animals, and vegetation in a geographic area. **Ecologic Studies** are used to study communities in certain geographic regions or time periods when individual exposure data is not available. Most often ecologic studies evaluate the effect of an exposure or an occupation on disease. They are primarily used to generate hypotheses.

Case Reports and Series are merely case descriptions of disease that are occurring, but they play an important role in linking clinical medicine

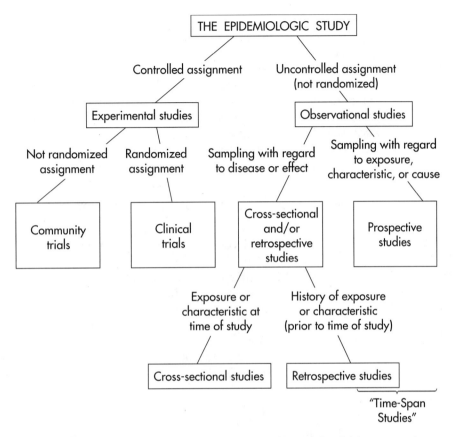

Fig. 5-1 A flow diagram of epidemiologic study. (From Lilienfield, A.M., and Lilienfield, D.E. 1980. Foundations of epidemiology. Second edition. Oxford University Press, New York.)

and the field of epidemiology. **Cross-Sectional Studies and Surveys** are quick and less difficult than some other types of studies and allow a look at both exposure and disease in individuals at the same time. Descriptive observational studies are a quick, easy, and inexpensive option to collecting important preliminary data about the cause of disease.

Analytic studies are designed to test hypotheses about the association of risk factors and disease. The design of the analytic study depends on whether the focus of interest is the exposure or the disease. **Prospective or Cohort Studies** are considered the "ideal" of the observational studies. These studies select individuals according to a particular exposure of interest. That is, these individuals have been exposed to a factor that is thought to cause disease. This group, along with a group that has not been exposed, is followed forward in time to see if they develop a disease. Because people must be followed forward in time, these studies are difficult, expensive, and may require years before useful data are obtained. An alternative is the case-control or retrospective study. **Case-Control Studies (Retrospective)** select cases of a defined disease and compare this group to a control group that is not diseased. Both groups, cases and controls, are followed back in time to look at their exposures. Because the events have already occurred, case-control studies are easier, quicker, and less expensive to do than prospective studies.

List of Principles

Natural, Ecologic Studies   Natural and ecologic studies are unique among observational studies. Natural experiments are rare occurrences of exposures that occur under natural conditions and allow the opportunity to study the possible causes of disease in that exposed group of individuals. Ecologic studies evaluate exposures and disease on a community level rather than an individual level. A community that has been exposed in a particular geographic area or has lived during a specific time period is evaluated.

Case Reports or Series   Case reports and series offer an important link between clinical medicine and epidemiology. Case reports give a clinical description of a patient or a group of patients (series) with an unusual disease or condition. These reports may be the first description of a new disease and offer important clues to the epidemiologist.

Cross-Sectional, Survey Studies   Cross-sectional studies measure both the exposure and disease in an individual or population at the same specific point in time. These studies can also explore the role of risk factors in the cause of a disease. Cross-sectional and survey studies offer a quick, easy, and inexpensive method of exploring the relationship between exposures and disease. These studies offer only a glimpse of the association between exposure and disease at one point in time so no definite conclusions about risk or cause can be made.

Prospective, Cohort Studies   Prospective studies follow individuals from the time of exposure to the time they develop disease. Prospective studies are the only observational studies that can measure incidence and give a clear idea of cause. A cohort is a group of individuals that have the same characteristic at a given time and are often used in prospective studies.

Case-Control, Retrospective Studies   Case-control studies can be done quickly, with limited expense and sample size, to determine the possible cause of a particular disease. Cases are selected on the basis of a particular disease of interest and evaluated back in time to determine the possible causes for the disease. Case-control studies cannot determine the incidence of disease; therefore they can only estimate risk of disease.

Natural, Ecologic Studies

Natural and ecologic studies are unique among observational studies. Natural experiments are rare occurrences of exposures that occur under natural conditions and allow the opportunity to study the possible causes of disease in the exposed group of individuals. Ecologic studies evaluate exposures and disease on a community level rather than an individual level. A community that has been exposed in a particular geographic area or has lived during a specific time period is evaluated.

Explanation

It is rare when an experiment of interest occurs naturally in the population, but "natural" experiments offer an unique opportunity to gain important information about disease and the association of variables to that disease. The classic example of a natural experiment is John Snow's discovery of cholera transmission through water. In the early 1850s Snow hypothesized that the increase in cases of cholera in London was due to cholera being transmitted in a water supply contaminated by fecal waste. During an outbreak in 1853, Snow determined that households receiving their water from one water company had almost an eightfold difference in mortality from cholera than households getting their water from another water company. The water company supplying the community with the highest death rates was getting its water from regions of the Thames River that were contaminated with sewage. Even before the causative organism was discovered, Snow had figured out the cause of cholera. This was 20 years before the development of the microscope! A more recent disaster example of a natural experiment is the nuclear radiation leak in Chernobyl, Russia. This unfortunate, tragic, leak has provided an on-going natural experiment on the short- and long-term effects of radiation in the environment, animals, and humans.

Ecologic studies are different from normal observational studies because, instead of collecting data on individuals, the focus is on collecting data on communities. They are called ecologic studies because the community of individuals live in a specific geographic area, such as a country, or live during a specified time period. The unit of comparison for the frequency of exposure and disease is the community or it can be a time period. That is, changes in an exposure during a period of time can be compared to changes in disease occurrence during a period of time for various population groups. Changes in exposure may be associated to changes in disease rates.

It is essential to remember that such a study does not collect exposure or outcome data on each individual but rather on the total number of individuals exposed and diseased within that community or time period. These total numbers for the exposure and for the disease are usually obtained from different sources that happen to be available for use. For example, cancer registries routinely collect data on the incidence of various cancers by geographic regions. At the same time, the Environmental Protection Agency often collects information about environmental pollutants by geographic area. Combining the information from both databases may help evaluate the effect of certain exposures on cancer incidence in a geographic area. But it also makes sense that if these two sources of data are collected independently, there is no way to conclude that the exposure data on one group is the same group for which the disease information is known. There is no information involving individuals. Therefore if an *assumption* is made that the association found on the community level is also true on the individual level, then a seriously biased conclusion, called an ecologic fallacy, will be committed.

These studies are useful for formulating hypotheses that can be further studied by analytic studies. Obviously they cannot be used to determine the cause of disease. For example, a lower incidence of coronary heart disease in Japan compared to the United States may help a hypothesis to be formulated about the culture and their diet. Ecologic studies are usually convenient because data are often available. Different state and federal agencies collect demographic data and reportable disease information. Medical insurance companies, such as Health Maintenance Organizations, collect data on disease and medical history. Different data sources can be used collectively to study the effect of risk factors on disease.

Examples

1. A current example of a natural experiment is a study of the acute and chronic effects on individuals exposed to burning crude oil. This is

possible by following over time the military personnel who were involved in the Persian Gulf War.

2. An example of an ecologic fallacy:

   Three countries, United States, Mexico, and Canada, are compared with respect to both television ownership and the annual incidence of brain cancer. The United States has the highest reported televisions per capita at 2.5, Canada is second with 1.8, and Mexico is third with 1.2. The annual incidence of brain cancer in the United States is 200 per 100,000; in Canada, it is 100 per 100,000; and in Mexico, 30 per 100,000. By looking at this data, one could conclude that watching television causes brain cancer. This assumption is obviously false. There is no information about whether the *individuals* who own the televisions are the ones who had brain cancer. Also, there are certain risk factors such as hereditary and injury factors for brain cancer that are not considered in these numbers.

3. Another example of a successful ecologic study:

   Data on driver education courses and fatal automobile accidents that involved teenage drivers were collected from 27 states. The information on the driver education courses was collected from the Insurance Institution on Highway Safety along with the National Safety Council. The automobile accident information was collected from police and motor vehicle administration records. Although conclusions on an individual level could not be done, an association was found. After controlling for possible confounding variables, such as speed limits and traffic patterns, this study found an association between driver education and the frequency of fatal crashes. This was due to the positive association of driver education and the increase in teenage drivers on the road.

TERMS

Ecologic Fallacy	An error or serious bias that occurs when associations seen in the populations studied are assumed to be also occurring at the individual level
Ecologic Study	A study of a group or population rather than an individual, usually on the basis of a geographic region or a time period
Natural Experiment	Naturally occurring events in a population that can be used as an experiment to make observations about risk factors and disease

Related Principles

Therapeutic versus intervention (Basic epidemiologic methodology)

Experimental versus observational (Basic epidemiologic methodology)

Information bias (Bias and error)

Person, place, and time (Epidemiologic concepts of disease)

Citation Classic

Snow, J. 1855. On the mode of communication of cholera. 2nd edition. Churchill Livingstone, London.

References

Firebaugh, G. 1978. A rule for inferring individual-level relationships from aggregate data. Am. Sociol. Rev. 43: 557-572.

Kelsey, J.L., Thompson, W.D., and Evans, A.S. 1986. Methods in observational epidemiology. Monographs in epidemiology and biostatistics. Vol 10. Oxford University Press, New York.

Morganstern, H. 1982. Uses of ecologic analysis in epidemiological research. Am. J. Public Health 72:1336-1344.

Robertson, L.S., Zador, P.L. 1978. Driver education and fatal crash involvement of teenage drivers. Am. J. Public Health 68:959-965.

Robinson, W.S. 1950. Ecologic correlations and the behavior of individuals. Am. Sociological Review 15: 351-357.

Case Reports or Series

Case reports and series offer an important link between clinical medicine and epidemiology. Case reports give a clinical description of a patient or a group of patients (series) with an unusual disease or condition. These reports may be the first description of a new disease and offer important clues to the epidemiologist.

Explanation

Case reports or series are most often published in medical journals such as the New England Journal of Medicine. Case reports are accounts of individual patients with an unexpected disease or medical event. Case series are accounts of a group of patients with the same medical condition. A case series is more useful than a single report for formulating a hypothesis because several patients provide more information and may represent a trend. The main advantage of case reports and series is that they present clinical information about a medical condition, perhaps for the first time. The clinical information includes the attributes of the patients involved, the duration of illness, and the place. Awareness about a new or unusual condition results in more reports and possible hypotheses about the cause. Case series and reports are often the beginning of the discovery of an important new disease or to a clue about an previously unknown risk factor for a disease.

Examples

1. In late 1980 and early 1981, 5 cases of *Pneumocystis carinii* pneumonia were reported in previously healthy young men in California. A short time later, Kaposi's sarcoma was reported in young homosexual men. Both of these conditions were unusual in that these diseases, before that time, were seen only in the elderly or severely immunocompromised individuals. This was the beginning of the discovery of the human immunodeficiency virus (HIV) and the acquired immunodeficiency disease syndrome (AIDS).
2. Spontaneous reports of adverse reactions to drugs and devices are scanned for clues of possible serious side effects to particular drugs and devices. It was the first clinical reports from England of serious congenital defects in babies whose mothers had taken thalidomide that triggered the hypothesis that thalidomide caused birth defects.

TERMS

Case Report	A report in the literature of a patient with an unusual medical event or disease
Case Series	A description of several patients with the same unique medical condition or event

Related Principles

Person, place, time (Epidemiologic concepts of disease)
Objective and hypothesis (Basic epidemiologic methodology)
Interdisciplinary (Overview)
Population medicine (Overview)

References

CDC. 1981. Kaposi's sarcoma and Pneumocystis pneumonia among homosexual men: New York City and California. MMWR. 30:305.
CDC. 1981. Pneumocystis pneumonia: Los Angeles. MMWR. 30:250.
Fletcher, R.H., Fletcher, S.W., and Wagner, E.H. 1982. Clinical epidemiology: the essentials. Williams & Wilkins. Baltimore, Maryland.
Lenz, W. 1962. Thalidomide and congenital abnormalities (Letters to the Editor) Lancet 1:45.
McBride, W.G. 1961. Thalidomide and congenital abnormalities (Letter to the Editor) Lancet 2:1358.

Cross-Sectional, Survey Studies

Cross-sectional studies measure both the exposure and disease in an individual or population at the same specific point in time. These studies can also explore the role of risk factors in the cause of a disease. Cross-sectional and survey studies offer a quick, easy, and inexpensive method of exploring the relationship between exposures and disease. These studies offer only a glimpse of the association between exposure and disease at one point in time so no definite conclusions about risk or cause can be made.

Explanation

Cross-sectional studies and surveys are also considered descriptive. The term *cross-sectional study* refers to the fact that this method measures the exposure and disease at the same point in time. That is, the study is a "cross-sectional" picture of the population at a specified time. Because an individual's exposure and disease status are examined at the same point in time, it is unclear which came first. Thus only the prevalence of disease can be determined, not the incidence. Cross-sectional studies are often called prevalence studies. The time studied may be a certain defined period of time or more often a fixed point in time. Cross-sectional studies include serologic studies, some ecologic studies, some acute epidemic investigations, and surveys. These studies can provide important information about the potential for associations between exposures and disease. It is important to remember that since there is no way to determine whether the association came before the disease, no conclusions about risk or cause can be made.

Cross-sectional studies can also provide data about the frequency and distribution of disease and other variables of interest in a population. The United States Census is done every four years to collect demographic data on the United States population. In addition, the National Center for Health Statistics conducts different focused surveys within the United States every few years, such as the National Health and Nutrition Examination Survey (NHANES) or the National Health Interview Survey (NHIS), to answer specific questions about health and disease.

The fact that one point in time is studied has advantages and disadvantages. The advantages are that the study can be accomplished fairly quickly, easily, and with minimal expense. It is an easy and quick way to determine possible associations about risk factors and a disease; therefore cross-sectional studies are often used in an acute outbreak of illness to determine possible causes. The disadvantage of the cross-sectional approach is that the study only offers a "snapshot" of time and of the population. The disease of interest may be disproportionately selected, or not selected, in the sampled population. This is especially true if studying a chronic disease. If the population was sampled during a time when more than a few individuals were in remission, then the number of actual diseased individuals or prevalence of the disease would be underestimated. Conversely, if the cross-sectional sample is taken during the later part of the disease and the disease was influenced by some factor that increases the survival of an individual with that disease, the affected population is oversampled.

Surveys are commonly used cross-sectional studies. Surveys can be done by different methods: self-administered, mailed, telephone interviews, face-to-face interviews, and even by computers. Each have advantages and disadvantages. Self-administered and computer interviews are good for sensitive information. Training is needed for interviewers doing face-to-face or telephone surveys to standardize the process and prevent the interviewers from subconsciously soliciting biased information. The response rate can be extremely low, 30% to 60%, for mail-in surveys, although they are the easiest to do. The low response rate must be taken into consideration when calculating the sample size needed to give sufficient power for the study. Consideration must also be given to the fact that some groups of individuals are more likely to respond than others.

There are two crucial methodological issues in conducting a survey, the questionnaire design and the sampling strategy. The types of questions asked determine what information is collected. Open-ended questions invite the respondent to fill in information. Although this information is interesting to read and may give additional information, it is difficult to quantify and analyze and may not address the hypothesis. Close-ended questions give answers for the respondents to choose from. For example, the answers may be yes or no or may be a multiple choice question. Close-ended questions allow the responses to be measured equally among all respondents. It is wise to do pilot testing of the questionnaire to see if the questions are worded clearly and that participants understand the question as the researcher intends. Pilot testing involves administering the questionnaire to a small sample of individuals to test whether the questionnaire is interpreted correctly and whether the questionnaire collects the information needed for the study.

The sampling plan is also important for a valid study to get a representative sample of the population of interest. In part, the sampling plan depends on what research question is asked and what part of the population needs to be sampled. The different approaches include random, stratified, clustered, and multiple stages.

Random sampling is when each person has the same opportunity to be selected. The sampling is often done with a computer or a random numbers table. The random numbers table picks a number, and the individual that is identified by that number is selected. The process is repeated. Stratified sampling is done by dividing the population into strata or groups with a characteristic of interest. Then individuals are selected randomly within each strata. Stratified sampling is commonly used and allows the sample within the designated strata to be representative of the total population in regard to a certain characteristic of interest. Cluster sampling involves sampling clusters or units of individuals. Then individuals within the clusters are evaluated. For example, schools are sampled as units, rather than each individual school child, to evaluate the frequency of vaccination and preventable diseases. A cluster sample is not homogeneous but is often used in national surveys. If there are multiple research questions, multiple stage sampling is used. Multiple stage sampling is done by taking samples at different stages. For example, the first sampling could be a city. The second stage could be city blocks, and the third stage could be individual households.

Examples

1. A serologic survey of hepatitis antibodies is done on new military recruits. A blood sample is drawn at the time of entering into the military; antibody titers for hepatitis are measured. The blood can also be frozen and used for comparison to a later sampling of the same group to see if the antibody levels have changed.
2. A random sample is generated of family practitioners in the United States. A 20% sample of these practitioners is mailed a questionnaire asking about auditory thermometer use in medical offices as opposed to the standard thermometers. The questionnaire asks about the use of the thermometer, the model used, and the perceptions of the respondents about accuracy and precision.

TERMS

Cross-Sectional Study	A study that looks at the relationship between disease and exposure at the same time it is occurring in the population
Questionnaire	A specific set of questions designed to collect data for a survey
Survey	A study in which data are systematically collected with a questionnaire or data form

Related Principles
Sample size (Basic epidemiologic methodology)
Experimental versus observational (Basic epidemiologic methodology)
Incidence, prevalence (Measures of frequency and association)
Selection bias (Bias and error)
Information bias (Bias and error)

References
Checkoway, H., Pearce N.E., and Crawford-Brown, D.J. 1989. Research methods in occupational epidemiology. Monographs in epidemiology and biostatistics. Vol 13. Oxford University Press, New York.

Dillman, D.A. 1978. Mail and telephone surveys: the total design method. John Wiley, New York.

Fowler, F.J. 1984. Survey research methods. Applied social research methods series, Vol 1. Sage Publications. Beverly Hills, California.

Groves, R.M., and Kahn, R.L. 1979. Surveys by telephone: a national comparison with personal interviews. Academic Press, New York.

Kelsey, J.L., Thompson, W.D., and Evans, A.S. 1986. Methods in observational epidemiology. Monographs in epidemiology and biostatistics. Vol 10. Oxford University Press, New York.

Waksberg, J. 1978. Sampling methods for random digit dialing. J. of Am. Stat. Assoc. 73: 40-66.

Prospective, Cohort Study

Prospective studies follow individuals from the time of exposure to the time they develop disease. Prospective studies are the only observational studies that can measure incidence and give a clear idea of cause. A cohort is a group of individuals that have the same characteristic at a given time and is often used in prospective studies.

Explanation

Among observational studies, the prospective study is considered the most rigorous scientifically because it can measure disease incidence and, consequently, estimate risk of disease resulting from a particular exposure. The prospective study selects individuals on the basis of an exposure of interest and follows them forward in time to measure the incidence of outcome or disease. The exposure of interest is usually selected because there is already some evidence of an association between that particular factor and the disease.

The first step in a prospective study is to select an existing cohort or group of individuals that would be appropriate for the study of the exposure or risk factor of interest. This cohort is then divided into groups of those that are exposed and those that are not exposed, or those with a risk factor and those without a risk factor. A cohort is a group of individuals that share a common experience within a defined time period. For example, members of a birth cohort are all born the same year or a period of years, whereas an occupational cohort are all hired at the same time or have the same profession. This group or cohort is followed forward in time until they develop disease. Cohorts can be used in prospective or retrospective studies, although they are most often used in the former.

The selection of the cohort is important. For example, when studying infectious disease, it is vital to determine who is susceptible and who is immune. If individuals are immune, they are not at risk of developing disease. It is also important for the cohort to be classified correctly as to whether they have been exposed or not and the amount of time of exposure. In occupational studies, the number of years of exposure is a simple surrogate for dose. Those exposed are supposed to be representative, with the exception of the exposure, of the general population in respect to their risk of disease. Both the exposed and the nonexposed group must have the same risk of developing disease outside of the exposure. For example, the comparison of a group of police officers who walk on their shift and a group of police officers who ride all day to evaluate the risk of heart attacks would not be appropriate. Those police officers walking would get much more exercise, which decreases the risk of a heart attack. The endpoint or outcome must be clearly defined. If the outcome is a disease, then the diagnostic criteria or definition must also be clearly defined.

Prospective studies can measure incidence because the exposed individuals are followed until they develop the disease or become a new case. The ability to measure incidence enables estimates of risk such as relative risk and attributable risk. Although subjects are selected on the basis of exposure or a risk factor of interest, the real issue of interest is the outcome. By selecting the exposure and following it forward in time, multiple outcomes can be studied. Rare exposures, *not* diseases, can also be studied because exposure is the starting point. Rare exposures would be difficult to find in old employee records. Finally, because there is a temporal sequence from cause to effect, prospective studies can establish causation.

Prospective studies require a large sample size, a long duration before the results are known, and a large amount of work and money to complete. The large sample size is needed to obtain enough individuals with and without the risk factor to follow, especially since some individuals will drop out of the study over time. These extensive requirements often limit the use of prospective studies. The most common use of prospective studies is to prove a suspected association found in other preliminary studies such as a cross-sectional study or survey.

There are also disadvantages with prospective studies because of the time required to complete them. One important disadvantage to following a cohort over time is the follow-up itself. Without follow-up of the entire cohort, there will be no information about the incidence of disease in those individuals. The number that may be lost to follow-up must also be considered when determining the required sample size for the study. The duration of the follow-up period varies with the disease and the resources available. The follow-up may involve periodic health exams, blood sampling, medical or hospital review, or even the documentation of deaths through death certificates. Occupational studies of mortality may be easier to accomplish because the important information is already collected and available. Employers normally have good records of individual work histories. In addition, many employers require preemployment physical examinations and periodic check-ups thereafter. Work histories usually include absences resulting from sickness, injury, or disability.

Individuals that are lost to follow-up require effort to find. It is important to find out as much as possible about those that are lost to follow-up to see if there are any differences from those individuals still in the studies. Differences between the groups not related to the exposure can give inaccurate results. Other factors that are relevant over time are whether diagnostic procedures or treatments change or whether individuals from one group (without exposure) may change to the other group and become exposed.

One option to avoid the disadvantages of a prospective study is to select the cohort with the exposure of interest from past records of exposure and then follow to the present to observe the outcome. This is often called a historical prospective or historical cohort study. This study can still measure incidence because the temporal sequence is established from exposure to disease. The advantage is that some of the time has already lapsed and a faster result is achieved. The problem with this method is making sure that records can be found for the cohort of exposed and unexposed and that the important information is available and not missing from the records.

Like any other study designs, the exposed and unexposed groups need to be comparable so that the only differences in incidence are due to the factor being studied. If study design can not produce groups that are comparable, statistical analysis (regression) can be used to account for differences in the groups.

Examples

1. Nurses Health Study: In the United States 120,000 female nurses were enrolled, beginning in 1976, in an ongoing cohort study to eval-

uate the effects of oral contraceptives on disease. The nurses were married, ages 30 to 55 years, and lived in 11 different states. Each nurse completed a questionnaire asking about medical and reproductive history, demographic information, and lifestyle. There is a two year follow-up of the original information, any disease event, and other variables of interest. This cohort study has provided data on the use of oral contraception and the risk of breast and ovarian cancer and myocardial infarction. These data have been and will continue to be used to evaluate other diseases as well.

2. Framingham Heart Study was started in 1949. It is a prospective cohort study that has followed residents of Framingham, Massachusetts, for over 30 years to look at risk factors for coronary heart disease. The starting cohort did not include anyone under 30 years of age because the risk of heart disease would be minimal over the next 10 to 20 years. Baseline measurements of cholesterol and blood pressure levels, smoking habits, and other factors were taken at the beginning of the study. Residents were followed and the incidence of coronary heart disease was recorded. Periodic measurements were taken of the cholesterol and blood pressure levels and other factors. This study was the first to show definitively that increased cholesterol and blood pressure could predict coronary heart disease. This cohort study has also provided the opportunity to study the role of risk factors in other diseases such as cancer and strokes.

TERMS

Cohort   A group of individuals having a common characteristic at the same specified time period

Historical Cohort A cohort study accomplished by selecting the cohort with the exposure of interest from past records and following the individuals to the present to determine the disease incidence

Prospective   Follow forward in time

Related Principles
Incidence, prevalence (Measures of frequency and association)
Relative risk (Measures of frequency and association)
Attributable risk (Measures of frequency and association)
Causation (Causality)
Cross-sectional, survey studies

References

Belanger, C.F., Hennekens, C.H., Rosner, R. et al. 1978. The nurses' health study. Am. J. Nurs. 78:1039.

Breslow, N.E., and Day, N.E. 1987. Statistical methods in cancer research II: the design and analysis of cohort studies. International Agency for Research in Cancer. Lyons, France.

Dawber, T.R. 1980. The Framingham study: the epidemiology of athero-sclerotic disease. Harvard University Press. Cambridge, Massachusetts.

Dawber, T.R., Meadors, G.F, and Moore, Jr., F.E. 1951. Epidemiological approaches to heart disease: the Framingham Study. Am. J. Public Health 41: 279-286.

Dawber, T.R., Kannel, W.B. and Lyell, L.P. 1963. An approach to longi-tudinal studies in a community: The Framingham Study. Ann. N.Y. Acad. Sci. 107:539-556.

Dawber, T.R., Moore, F.E., and Mann, G.V. II. 1957. Coronary heart disease in the Framingham Study. Am. J. Public Health 47:4-24.

Kannel, W.B., and Abbott, R.D. 1984. Incidence and prognosis of unrec-ognized myocardial infarction. An update on the Framingham study. N. Engl. J. Med. 311:1144-1147.

Kannel, W.B., Dawber, T.R., Kagan, A. et al. 1961. Factors of risk in the development of coronary heart disease: six year follow-up experience: The Framingham Study. Ann. Int. Med. 55:33-50.

Kleinbaum, D.G., and Kupper, L.L. 1978. Applied regression analysis and Other multivariable methods. Duxbury Press. North Scituate, Massachusetts.

Case-Control, Retrospective Study

Case-control studies can be done quickly, with limited expense and sample size, to determine the possible cause of a particular disease. Cases are selected on the basis of a particular disease of interest and evaluated back in time to determine the possible causes for the disease. Case-control studies cannot determine the incidence of disease; therefore they can only estimate risk of disease.

Explanation

Case-control studies are differentiated from the other analytic type of study, prospective or cohort, by two important facts. Cases are selected on the basis of disease not exposure. The study goes back in time to look for the exposures or risk factors of interest and therefore can only mea-sure prevalent cases.

The proper selection of cases and controls is a key component to the design and success of the case-control study. The criteria for the selection of cases and controls should be equal. Both cases and controls must have the same opportunity for the exposure of interest. Cases are selected on the basis of the disease of interest. The control group (without disease) is used to compare with the cases in regards to the exposure. Sources for case selection are hospital or outpatient admissions, disease registries, and even insurance or Medicare records. When possible, controls should also be selected from the same population. For example, controls can be selected from the hospital population that the cases were chosen from. However, the controls must not have the same or similar disease as the cases. In some instances, the controls may be selected from the local community or geographic area, or even friends and relatives. It is important that controls and cases be comparable, except for the disease, so that other differences are not introduced that affect the results. For example, hospital patients are sicker than the general population, and certain diseases are overrepresented in the hospital population. If a factor being studied also affects the disease in the controls, a true association may be masked or an association that is not really true may be found.

The primary role for the controls is to give an estimate of the rate of exposure that would occur in the cases assuming that there was no association between the disease and exposure of interest. Matching of controls, or pairing of one or more controls to a case on the basis of a similar variable, is sometimes done to increase the power of the study without having to increase the sample size. Primarily, matching is done to ensure that cases and controls are comparable. It is important to ensure that the variable on which the cases and controls are matched is independent of the exposure and not a variable to be studied. Matching on a variable prevents the study of its effect on the disease. If matching is done, the statistical analysis must take the matched design into account.

Case-control studies are often termed *retrospective studies* because they go back in time to determine the exposure; case-control studies start with the effect and attempt to determine the cause. Because only prevalence is measured, the odds ratios can only estimate risk. If the disease studied is rare, however, then the odds ratio is an approximation of the relative risk. The important concept to remember is that even though the case-control study starts with the selection of cases on the basis of their disease, the primary objective is to study the hypothesis about the cause or exposure. Case-control studies can look at *multiple exposures but only one effect.*

The disadvantages of retrospective studies are that the records used to collect the information may be incomplete and there may be no method of obtaining the needed data. If respondents are required to recall information or events, the recall may not be accurate or complete; it may even be biased. Serious illnesses are more easily remembered than minor ones.

Case-control studies have been less respected scientifically than the prospective cohort studies but they are gaining wide acceptance in the epidemiology community when properly designed and carried out. These studies offer the advantage of being able to do rigorous studies quickly and with limited expense and a reasonable sample size. They are especially useful for the study of rare diseases or exposures that normally would require a large sample size. They are also useful for studying chronic or latent diseases that would take years from the time of exposure to the onset of disease before any data could be collected.

Examples

1. A historical example of a case-control study is the discovery that the taking of diethylstilbestrol in pregnant women causes vaginal cancer in their daughters. Between 1966 and 1969, there were reports of seven women between the ages of 15 and 22 years being diagnosed with vaginal adenocarcinoma. This cancer is rare in women younger than 50 years of age. Because of these reports, a study was initiated to determine the cause of this cancer in young women. A case-control study design was appropriate because the cancer is a rare occurrence. In addition, the time period from exposure to event is too long to be studied prospectively.

   Four controls for each patient were selected that were the same age as the cases (within 5 days). Interviews of the mothers of the cases and controls were done and a variety of factors evaluated. None of the controls had mothers who had taken estrogen while pregnant. All but one of the mothers of the cases had taken estrogen while pregnant. There were no other differences in variables.

2. An increase in fibrosarcomas in cats was reported starting in 1991. The fibrosarcomas occurred subcutaneously. Studies were initiated to determine the cause of the increase and the presence of the fibrosarcoma in the subcutaneous tissue. Retrospective studies collected cases from veterinary pathology diagnostic laboratories and extracted vaccination history information from medical records. Various factors such as vaccination history, injury, and other medical conditions were evaluated. The only common exposure that was found among the cases was that of a rabies vaccination given subcutaneously in the previous year. Although rabies vaccines were originally thought to be the only cause, a history of other vaccinations also shows an increased risk (e.g., Feline Leukemia vaccine). The additives used in the vaccines are being examined to see if they are the direct cause of the reaction. This study in animals may be useful for causes of sarcoma in humans as well.

TERMS

Case-Control	A study that selects cases that have a disease of interest, a comparable control (without disease) group, and goes back in time to examine the exposure
Matching	The pairing of one or more controls to a case on the basis of some variable of interest that is not related to the exposure
Retrospective	Going back in time

Related Principles
Odds ratio (Measures of frequency and association)
Incidence, prevalence (Measures of frequency and association)
Prospective, cohort study

Citation Classics
Cole, P. 1979. The evolving case-control study. J. Chronic Dis. 32: 15-34.
Cornfield, J. 1951. A method of estimating comparative rates from clinical data. Applications to cancer of the lung, breast, and cervix. J. of National Cancer Inst. 11:1269-1275.
Mantel, N., and Haenszel, W. 1959. Statistical aspects of the analysis of data from retrospective studies of disease. J. National Cancer Inst. 22:719-748.
Schlesselman, J.J. 1982. Case-control studies: design, conduct, analysis. Monographs in epidemiology and biostatistics, Vol 2. Oxford University Press, New York.

References
Breslow, N. 1982. Design and analysis of case-control studies. Ann. Rev. Pub. Health 3: 29-54.
Breslow, N.E., and Day, N.E. 1980. Statistical methods in cancer research. Vol 1. The analysis of case-control studies. International Agency for Research on Cancer. Lyons, France.
Herbst, A.L., Hubby, M.M., Blough, R.R., and Azizi, F. 1980. A comparison of pregnancy experience in DES-exposed and DES-unexposed daughters. J. Reproduc. Med. 24:62-69.
Herbst A.L., Ulfelder, H., and Poskanzer, D.C. 1971. Adenocarcinoma of the vagina. Association of maternal stilbestrol therapy with tumor appearance in young women. New England J. of Med. 284:878-881.
Ibrahim, M.A., (ed.). 1979. Case-control study: consensus and controversy. J. Chronic Dis. 32:1-144.

Kelsey, J.L., Thompson, W.D., Evans, A.S. 1986. Methods in observational epidemiology. Monographs in epidemiology and biostatistics. Vol 10. Oxford University Press, New York.

Lane-Claypon, J.E. 1926. A further report on cancer of the breast. Rept. Publ Hlth. Med. Subj. 32. London. HMSO.

Lilienfeld, A.M., and Lilienfeld, D. 1979. A century of case-control studies-progress. J. Chron. Dis. 32:5-13.

West, D.W., Schuman, K.L., Lyon, J.L., Robison, L.M., and Allred, R. 1984. Differences in risk estimations from a hospital and a population-based case control study. Int. J. of Epidemiol. 13:235-239.

Observational Studies: Study Questions

1. Explain the differences between case-control and cohort studies.
2. Give the advantages and disadvantages of both case-control and cohort studies.
3. What characteristic makes ecologic studies unique? What about this characteristic would also make conclusions resulting from ecologic studies more "dangerous"?
4. Describe a natural experiment (other than mentioned in the text) that has occurred and the possible information that might be gained.
5. Justify the importance of case reports being published in medical journals. Give an example of a case series and describe how you would take the information given and study it further. What hypotheses can be formulated?
6. Explain why you cannot make generalizations or conclude causation from the results of cross-sectional studies.
7. Describe a study that would be appropriately studied through the survey method. What would be the most appropriate method of survey for this study: mail-in, face-to-face, telephone, computer, and why? What are the advantages and disadvantages of each?
8. Explain each type and the appropriate circumstances for using each sampling scheme: random, stratified, cluster, multistage.
9. What is the best method to study the cause of a rare disease?
10. What is the best method to study a particular cancer?
11. Explain a historical cohort study.
12. Give examples of a disease or a problem that would be studied most effectively using a prospective study design. Give examples of a disease or a problem most effectively studied with the retrospective study.
13. Explain the influence or role of time in the cross-sectional, prospective, and retrospective methods.

14. Explain the importance of selecting the cohort for a prospective study.
15. Why cannot a retrospective study be used to calculate incidence?
16. Explain the importance of the selection of the controls in a case-control study.
17. What are the advantages and disadvantages of the method of matching?

CHAPTER 6

Bias and Error

The final step in any study is to draw conclusions from the data. Unless the conclusions about the sample population are accurate and, in some way, can be applied to the more general population, the study and the results are useless. An erroneous conclusion based on biased information can be worse than no conclusion at all because it may focus further study in the wrong direction. All experimental and observational studies involve the potential for error. One of the roles of an epidemiologist is to prevent or at least explain as much of the bias in a study as possible.

Error is the wrong assumption or conclusion. Random error occurs because of chance and cannot be predicted. Most random error that can be predicted or determined is due to sampling error. In other words, the sampling of the population is not representative and not probabilistic. The result of nonrandom sampling makes it impossible to generalize the conclusions to the general population. Systematic error is different from random error or chance. A consistent error such as the malfunction of a measurement device is considered systematic error or bias. The source of systematic error can usually be determined.

Bias can fall into three main categories depending on how it is introduced in the study: selection, information, and confounding. **Selection Bias** occurs when the selection of the study subjects is biased. This bias generally occurs at the start of a study. For example, self-selection bias can occur when people volunteer for a study or choose to fill out a questionnaire. Usually those individuals who volunteer for a study have a particular interest in the subject; this interest may influence the results. Sampling from populations of hospital patients, or even healthy workers, introduces certain biases related to that population. Hospital patients are sicker than the general population. Individuals who are able to work are obviously healthier than a group that includes an elderly or disabled population. If these populations are selected for a study where the bias is related to the hypothesis, incorrect conclusions are likely. A comparison, for example, of a working population with a retired population to study the incidence of cancer may give a biased result because those individuals able to work are not likely to have a disease, especially cancer. On the other hand, individuals that have retired are older and have a higher risk of cancer.

Information Bias is caused by the incomplete or inaccurate collection of data or observational outcomes. Such data may occur because the recall of past events is difficult, especially if a lot of time has passed. Subjects with serious illnesses are more likely than healthy individuals to remember past events that might have been associated with illness. In such a case, it cannot be concluded that the healthier individuals were not exposed just because they cannot recall the event. The most important type of information bias is misclassification. Because of incomplete or incorrect information, study subjects may be placed in the wrong group or "misclassified." This causes the number of individuals in each group to be incorrect and calculations, such as the relative risk, to be inaccurate.

Confounding is one of the most difficult biases to detect and control. Confounding is the distortion or the masking of an association between an exposure and an outcome because of a third extraneous factor. The presence of a third factor (other than exposure or outcome) is not enough to be considered confounding; there are often multiple factors in the causation of disease. The important point to remember is that this extraneous factor *has to be associated with the exposure* and also *has to be a direct risk factor for the disease.*

List of Principles

Error Error occurs when an incorrect assumption or conclusion is made about data. Error that occurs by chance is considered random error; most random error is due to incorrect sampling procedures. Error that occurs consistently is considered systematic error or bias; bias is a form of error.

Selection Bias Bias is the systematic error or distortion that results in an association between variables. Selection bias occurs when the selection of the study population for a certain disease in a case-control study is somehow related to the exposure history. Likewise, selection bias occurs in cohort studies when the selection of the cohort for an exposure is somehow related to the disease.

Information Bias   Information bias is a form of systematic error that occurs because the data that are collected or observed are incomplete or incorrect. Misclassification bias is the most serious form and occurs when cases are placed incorrectly in the noncase group and noncases are placed incorrectly in the case group.

Confounding   Confounding is the distortion or the masking of an association between an exposure and an outcome because of a third extraneous factor. The extraneous variable must be associated with the exposure and is also independently a risk factor for the disease.

Error

Error occurs when an incorrect assumption or conclusion is made about data. Error that occurs by chance is considered random error; most random error is due to incorrect sampling procedures. Error that occurs consistently is considered systematic error or bias; bias is a form of error.

Explanation

Error involves making the wrong assumption or conclusion about the data. Random error is what occurs by chance and cannot be predicted. When estimating random error, it is everything that is not considered systematic error. Systematic error occurs consistently, such as the faulty measurement of a testing device. Most random error is due to sampling error; that is, the sampling design of the study introduces error. For example, the sampling procedure may exclude some individuals that were important in the study of a particular exposure or disease. It is important in the sampling process that all individuals have the same opportunity to be sampled, or the sample will not be considered representative or valid. The size and design of a sample, as well as the distribution of the variable of interest, determines the sampling error. As random error increases, the precision of the study decreases. Random error can be decreased by increasing sample size or by making the study design more efficient so that the sample is representative.

Systematic error includes selection and information bias and confounding. As systematic error increases, the validity of the study decreases. Reduction of bias and confounding can only be achieved through good study design. Once bias is introduced into a study, it is difficult to correct the effects analytically.

Example

A telephone survey is designed to determine the frequency of healthcare usage in a given metropolitan area. The survey is conducted by randomly selecting phone numbers from the local telephone book to be interviewed. The subjects are asked about the frequency of doctor visits, visits to outpatient clinics, and visits to emergency clinics. Income and access to healthcare are two factors that influence the use of healthcare. Individuals without phones are more likely to have a lower income and to be more isolated in outlying areas. Therefore a sample of only those individuals with telephones could lead to an erroneous assumption.

TERMS

Error	An incorrect assumption or conclusion
Random Error	Error that occurs by chance
Precision	How well-defined or stated. The lack of random error
Validity	How well the sample results can be generalized to the true population or show a causal effect

Related Principles
Cross-sectional, survey studies (Observational studies)
Selection bias
Information bias

References
Fowler, F.J. 1984. Survey research methods: applied social research methods series, Vol 1. Sage Publications. Beverly Hills, California.
Levy, P.S., and Lemeshow, S. 1980. Sampling for health professionals. Lifetime Learning Publications. Belmont, California.

Selection Bias

Bias is the systematic error or distortion that results in an association between variables. Selection bias occurs when the selection of the study population for a certain disease in a case-control study is somehow related to the exposure history. Likewise, selection bias occurs in cohort studies when the selection of the cohort for an exposure is somehow related to the disease.

Explanation

Bias, in general, refers to the *systematic* distortion of the association between variables. It may also be termed *systematic error.* Bias occurs in situations when the introduction of information into the design or implementation of a study causes a spurious or masked association between the variables studied. Ideally, the design of the study should eliminate as much bias as possible. No study can completely eliminate bias; hence, it is essential to be aware of the potential for its presence and influence. The biased value (of the measure of association or risk) can either be closer or further away from the true population value.

Selection bias may occur in different ways depending on the study design and studied population. Selection bias occurs most often in case-control studies because the exposure and the disease have already occurred when the subjects are selected. The time of exposure is unknown, which makes it easier for the subjects to be selected by a disease that is somehow related to the exposure history. Bias can occur in the identification of cases when the selection of a specific disease somehow is dependent on the exposure that is going to be studied. For example, shipyard workers are selected as cases because they have a high rate of mesothelioma, a specific type of lung cancer. The reason, however, shipyard workers have a higher rate of mesothelioma is that their occupation involves large exposures to the cause of mesothelioma, which is asbestos. Similarly, if the exposure in the controls is somehow dependent on the disease of interest, there is selection bias. Selection bias distorts the effect measured.

Self-selection bias occurs when individuals refer themselves for treatment or volunteer for a study. Often the reason that the individuals volunteer is related to the study question. Individuals who are highly motivated to lose weight would be more likely than others to volunteer to participate in study that involved new behavioral techniques for modifying diet and exercise habits. Nonresponse in a survey also forms a population that is self-selected; those that choose to respond are self-selected. Nonresponse is an important issue to deal with in any type of survey whether it is a mail, telephone, or even personal interview. Response rates depend on the education and economic level of the respondent and whether the individuals responding to the surveys are interested in the topic. Those individuals with higher education and economic levels usually have higher response rates. Individuals living in rural areas have different response rates than those living in urban areas. The conclusions of the study can depend on those individuals that choose to respond and will be biased by the factors that make the individuals more likely to respond.

The healthy-worker effect is a form of self-selection bias that occurs in occupational studies. The actual self-selection occurs naturally and before the individuals are even selected. The healthy-worker effect is a bias that occurs when a comparison is made between a group of individuals selected from an occupation and a group of individuals selected from the general population. Those in the occupational group have a lower risk of mortality and morbidity. This is due to the fact that the workplace usually consists of individuals that are healthier than the general population and not necessarily because of the exposure studied. Those individuals in the general population who are not working at the time of the study may be healthy and unemployed or retired. They are also more likely to be individuals who are unable to work because of sickness or disability. It makes sense that older workers increase the healthy worker effect because the older an individual gets the less likely they are to work unless they are healthy. In general, younger workers have fewer health problems. This bias must be considered, especially when making comparisons of mortality rates between two groups with different work experience.

Lead-time bias is a type of bias that occurs in screening programs. It occurs because most diseases would become evident over time whether or not they are screened. The lead-time interval is the period of time between the detection of the condition through screening and the time it would have been clinically apparent by the symptoms. In this case, screening for the disease only allows diagnosis to occur more quickly; consequently, medical intervention may either cure or slow the progression of the disease. Earlier detection of a disease may or may not have an actual effect on the survival or mortality rate. Consideration must be given as to whether there is an effect, whether the effect is due to the diagnosed group being treated, or whether the effect is due to the detection of the disease occurring earlier.

Berkson's bias was first described in the 1940s and refers to the selection bias associated with the selection of study groups from hospital patient populations. Hospital patients are not representative of a healthy, general population and the reason for hospitalization may be associated with the exposure being studied in a case-control study. As a result of such bias, a study may conclude that there is an association between an exposure and disease because the control group has a different risk of exposure than the general population. For example, a person with more than one disease is more likely to be hospitalized and more at risk of disease than an individual that is healthy. Also, some diseases are more likely to result in hospitalization.

With the potential for Berkson's bias, why use hospital patients for a study population? If the cases are from a hospital population, it makes sense to select the controls from the hospital population as well, though they may be biased. It is easier to find individuals for inclusion into a control group, easier to evaluate or interview the individual, and easier to find the medical records. The biases between the groups will be similar. There are several options to prevent the bias when using a hospital population. One is to use several groups of controls within the hospital; therefore the differences will even out. Another common option is to select patient controls from disease diagnoses that are unrelated to the disease and the exposure of interest.

Examples
1. Healthy-Worker Effect
A case-control study of the risk of cancer of the reproductive organs resulting from exposure to ethylene oxide and other chemicals is done in a population of practicing veterinarians. The comparison group is residents of a retirement community. Cancer is more common in the elderly population. Also, those individuals working are less likely to have a serious form of cancer. Therefore, even if the chemicals did cause an increased risk of cancer in veterinarians, the effect would be diluted because only working, healthy veterinarians are being studied (fewer cases of cancer), and the number of cases in an elderly population would be higher just because the population is older, not because of any exposure.
2. Lead-Time Bias
A new screening test has been developed to detect early or subclinical prostate cancer in the formative stages. A study is done to compare the mortality rates of men with prostate cancer that have been diagnosed in the previous year with the new screening test and men with symptoms of prostate cancer that were diagnosed after they sought medical attention. The mortality rate in the men diagnosed with the new screening test may be lower than the men with symptoms of prostate cancer because the screening test allowed early diagnosis of prostate cancer and treatment. Those men with symptoms resulting from the cancer would have the disease in later stages and have a poorer prognosis for survival.

3. Berkson's Bias

A case-control study is done to evaluate the association between leukemia and diagnostic radiation exposure. The cases are hospital patients that have been admitted to a particular hospital in the last year and were diagnosed with leukemia. Medical records are evaluated for radiologic procedures, and patients are interviewed about other diagnostic radiation exposure, such as radiologic procedures done at other hospitals or at doctor's offices. The control group is selected from the hospital patient population and matched on age. An association may be shown not because there is a relationship between diagnostic radiologic exposure and leukemia, but because the control group may have a higher risk of diagnostic radiologic procedures than the general population. This would be especially true if the control group consisted of seriously ill patients that have required numerous diagnostics over a period of time.

TERMS

Berkson's Bias	Bias that occurs when using a study population from the hospital
Bias	Systematic error resulting in a distorted conclusion or assumption
Healthy-Worker Effect	Bias that is caused by the fact that healthy individuals are the ones that are working. The morbidity or mortality rates are naturally lower than the general population
Lead-Time Bias	Bias that occurs when comparing survival rates between a group that is screened for a disease and a group that is not screened. The fact that the disease is detected earlier because of screening makes the survival look longer. This is due to the fact that the disease is diagnosed earlier
Lead-Time Interval	The interval from the time the disease is detected with screening to the time the disease would normally be detected through the patient's symptoms
Self-Selection Bias	Bias caused by a study population that "volunteers" for the research because of an interest that is connected to the outcome of the research

Related Principles

Screening (Surveillance)
Confounding
Information bias
Case-control, retrospective studies (Observational studies)
Cross-sectional, survey studies (Observational studies)
Prospective, cohort studies (Observational studies)

Classic Citation

Berkson, J. 1946. Limitations of the application of fourfold table analysis to hospital data. Biometrics. Bull. 2: 47-53.

References

Feinstein, A.R., Walter, S.D., and Horowitz, R.I. 1986. An analysis of Berkson's bias in case-control studies. J. Chron Dis. 39:495-504.

Flanders, W.D., Boyle, C.A., and Boring, J.R. 1989. Bias associated with differential hospitalization rates in incident case-control studies. J. Clin. Epidemiol. 42:395-401.

Hutchison, G.B., and Shapiro, S. 1968. Lead time gained by diagnostic screening for breast cancer. J. Nat. Cancer Inst. 41:665-681.

Morrison, A.S. 1982. The effects of early treatment, lead time, and length bias on the mortality experienced by cases detected by screening. Int. J. Epidemiol. 111: 261-267.

Sackett, D.L. 1979. Bias in analytic research. J. Chronic. Dis. 32: 51-63.

Sartwell, P.E, Masi, A.T., Arthes, F.G., et al. 1969. Thromboembolism and oral contraceptives: an epidemiologic case-control study. Am. J. Epidemiol. 90:365-380.

Shapiro, S., Goldberg, J.D., and Hutchison, G.B. 1974. Lead time in breast cancer detection and implications for periodicity of screening. Am. J. Epidemiol. 100:357-366.

Walter, S.D. 1980. Berkson's bias and its control in epidemiologic studies. J. Chron Dis. 33:721-725.

Information Bias

Information bias is a form of systematic error that occurs because the data that are collected or observed are incomplete or incorrect. Misclassification bias is the most serious form and occurs when cases are placed incorrectly in the noncase group and noncases are placed incorrectly in the case group.

Explanation

Information bias is also a systematic error, but it occurs in the collection of data or observation of outcomes. Types of information bias include recall, interviewer, loss to follow-up, and the most serious one, misclassification.

Recall bias is most common with case-control studies in which individuals are asked to recall events from the past. The longer the time lapse from the event to the time of the interview, the less likely the individuals are to recall the information needed. The recall may be incomplete or it may be biased. It makes sense that the more serious the event, such as hospitalization, the more likely the individual is to remember the details. Also, individuals that have been sick are more likely to think about and recall possible causes. Media coverage about a disease or risk factor and an individual's knowledge of the hypothesis also increases the amount and the quality of the recall. Individuals are more likely to remember those exposures they think are related to the disease than unknown factors.

Interviewer bias can occur, especially if interviewers are not blinded to the study hypothesis. Bias occurs when the interviewer consciously or unconsciously solicits selected information from an individual that might favor the hypothesis. If training of interviewers is not done and a standardized set of questions is not used for the interview, then interviewer bias is more likely to happen.

Another form of bias occurs because of loss to follow-up in cohort studies. When participants drop out of a cohort study or cannot be located, important data about those individuals are lost. The reasons for the individuals dropping out of the study or the loss to follow-up are important. Their absence from the remainder of the study may be due to death or illness otherwise contributed to the exposure or the disease. Also, their absence may be due to an important difference in the population and therefore prevent comparability of the cohorts. For example, those lost to follow-up may be younger and more mobile. This may be important if age is related to the question being studied. It is essential to try to obtain information about those lost to follow-up to ensure these biases do not occur.

Misclassification is the most serious information bias and occurs because of inaccurate information that has been reported or recorded. It can also occur during statistical analyses when categories of data are collapsed to achieve a larger sample size within strata. Misclassification occurs when cases and controls are placed in the wrong groups; that is, cases are classified as controls and controls are classified as cases. Misclassification can occur in any type of study, especially if there is self-reporting. Self-reporting, unless validated, can often be unreliable. Misclassification is also common in occupational studies where exposure is uncertain or not easily measured.

The effect of misclassification depends on whether it occurs randomly or whether it occurs nonrandomly. Differential misclassification is the more serious of the two and occurs when the misclassification is nonrandom. That is, both the exposure or disease classification are incorrect for an equal proportion of individuals in both the case and control groups. The assumption is that the misclassification effect is equal among the exposed and nonexposed groups. Usually, the misclassification effect causes the relative risk estimate to be underestimated. Because it is of equal proportions, nondifferential misclassification is less of a threat to the validity of a study and the resultant bias is always in an underestimation.

Nonrandom, or differential misclassification, is a more serious problem because the misclassification occurs differently among the case and control groups. The errors in classification are not independent of each other. For example, the error in selection of cases and controls for a specific study of a disease is not independent of the exposure. Likewise, error in selection of a cohort for a study of a particular exposure is not independent of the disease of interest. Therefore the bias can be in either direction and can cause an overestimate or underestimate of the true association. This type of bias is more difficult to estimate and is more of a threat to the validity of the study.

Examples

1. Nondifferential Misclassification (Random)

   This example shows how random misclassification can underestimate the relative risk of disease.

   a. Original data:

   DISEASE X

Exposure	Yes	No	Ratio
Yes	100	100	100/200
No	20	180	20/200

   Rate ratio = 0.5/0.1 = 5.0

   b. Partially misclassified:

   Notice that the misclassification occurs the same way in those individuals diagnosed with the disease and those without disease. Twenty individuals from the diseased and the nondiseased had their exposure missed.

   DISEASE X

Exposure	Yes	No	Ratio
Yes	80	80	80/160
No	40	200	40/240

Rate ratio = 0.5/0.16 = 3.1

c. Totally misclassified:
Note that the misclassification occurred both in the disease category and in the exposure category.

DISEASE X

Exposure	Yes	No	Ratio
Yes	80	120	80/200
No	40	160	40/200

Rate ratio = 0.40/0.20 = 2.0

2. **Differential Misclassification (Nonrandom)**
Smokers are more likely to seek medical attention about possible respiratory problems than nonsmokers. If medical attention is sought, emphysema is more likely to be diagnosed. Otherwise, emphysema is usually underreported and underdiagnosed. Therefore emphysema would be diagnosed more in smokers (differential misclassification), and the misclassification error would occur more frequently in nonsmokers. That is, nonsmokers would be classified in the group without disease, when in fact, they have the disease. This misclassification is more likely to happen in a study in which the subjects give medical histories rather than undergo a physical exam.

TERMS

Information Bias	Bias that occurs because of lacking or incorrect information or data
Interviewer Bias	Bias that occurs when an interviewer solicits data that is biased in some way
Loss to Follow-Up Bias	Bias that occurs because those individuals that drop out of a study are different from those that stay in the study
Misclassification	Putting cases and controls in the wrong category
Recall	The ability to remember events that happened in the past

Related Principles
Blinding (Basic epidemiologic methodology)
Selection bias

Cross-sectional, survey studies (Observational studies)
Prospective, cohort studies (Observational studies)
Case-control, retrospective studies (Observational studies)

References

Barron, B.A. 1977. The effects of misclassification on the estimation of relative risk. Biometrics. 33: 414-418.
Bross, I. 1954. Misclassification in 2 × 2 tables. Biometrics. 10: 478-486.
Copeland, K.T., Checkoway, H., McMichael, A.J., and Holbrook, R.H. 1977. Bias due to misclassification in the estimation of relative risk. Am. J. of Epidemiol. 105: 488-95.
Flegal, K.M., Brown, C., and Haas, J.D. 1986. The effects of exposure misclassification on estimates of relative risk. Am. J. of Epidemiol. 123: 736-751.
Gladen, B., and Rogan, W.J. 1979. Misclassification and the design of environmental studies. Am. J. Epidemiol. 109:609-616.
Greenland, S. 1980. The effect of misclassification in the presence of covariates. Am. J. Epidemiol. 112:564-569.

Confounding

Confounding is the distortion or the masking of an association between an exposure and an outcome because of a third extraneous factor. The extraneous variable must be associated with the exposure and is also independently a risk factor for the disease.

Explanation

Confounding is an important form of bias to account for in epidemiologic studies. Confounding is the distortion, or the masking, of an association or an effect between an exposure and an outcome, such as a disease or event, by another extraneous variable. In other words, variable A causes a disease and is also associated with variable B. This association may make it look like variable B causes the disease. Confounding can increase, decrease, or even change the direction of the estimated association between an exposure and outcome; thus the conclusion from the data is biased.

Confounders themselves are variables that are associated with, but not a consequence of, the exposure. They also can cause the disease of interest. Apart from the association with exposure, the confounder has an effect; therefore even in nonexposed individuals, the confounder is related to the risk of disease. The confounder is predictive of disease occurrence. Confounders are *not* variables that are intermediate steps in a causal pathway but rather direct risk factors of disease. Sometimes it is difficult to determine if a third factor (a factor other than the associated exposure and the outcome) is present, and if it is, whether it is a direct cause of the disease or a confounder. According to Rothman, there are three criteria for a variable to be a confounder: it must be a risk factor for disease; it must be associated with exposure; and it must not be an intermediate step in the causal pathway.

How *can* the presence of confounding be determined other than by carefully analyzing the conclusions and the biologic plausibility of the association? The first step is to always look at the statistics, such as the t-test or chi-square test, calculated in the analysis of the differences between the two groups being studied. If there is a significant difference statistically in the groups with and without the second variable (the one for which there is concern), there is a good chance that there is confounding. Another statistical method to look for confounding is to stratify by the variable and see if the relative risk changes. If confounding is present, the adjusted relative risk after stratification is much lower than the crude relative risk. This happens because, by adjusting for the confounder, the actual risk for disease resulting from the exposure is reduced. Statistically, the mixing effect of the variable being studied and the confounder has been separated.

Several options are available to control for confounding: matching, stratification, statistical analysis, or regression. Matching is done in case-control studies and involves removing the effect of the confounder by making the case group and the control group equivalent in regards to the confounder. Each case is matched with one or more controls according to a certain factor (confounder of interest) to make sure that cases and controls are comparable. Stratification can also reduce or remove the confounding effect. By stratifying the groups by the confounding effect, the exposure can be evaluated within those strata. Statistical analysis using regression techniques has the advantage of controlling for several variables simultaneously by statistically adjusting for the confounding. The advantage of the statistical approach is that it can be done at the end of the study and it allows analysis of a greater range of associations and relationships. This can also be a disadvantage because the analysis is done after the study is computed. Another disadvantage is that a larger sample is needed for regression analysis than for some of the simpler statistical analyses.

Example

Cigarette smoking and coffee drinking are associated, probably because they usually occur at the same time. There have been many studies on the effects of cigarette smoking and the risk of cancer and other disease. There has been an increasing number of hypotheses about the effects of coffee drinking.

Two proposed hypotheses about the health effects of coffee are:

1. Coffee drinking has been linked to pancreatic cancer.
2. Coffee drinking by the mother has been linked to low birthweight in the neonate.

Studies have been done to look at both hypotheses and the results have shown an association of coffee consumption and an increase in the risk of pancreatic cancer and low birthweight. There is, however, a concern about the association of cigarette smoking and coffee consumption and whether the cigarette smoking has an effect. A second analysis of the results by controlling for cigarette smoking, showed the risk for both pancreatic cancer and low birthweight decreased. This was especially true with low birthweight.

For the study of the effects of coffee on the risk of pancreatic cancer or low birthweights, cigarette smoking is a confounder because:

- cigarette smoking is associated with coffee drinking
- cigarette smoking is a direct risk factor for pancreatic cancer and for low birthweight in the neonate
- cigarette smoking is not an intermediate step in the causal pathway of cigarette smoking causing cancer or low birthweight.
(According to Rothman's three criteria.)

TERMS

Confounder	A variable that is associated with the exposure and at the same time, is an independent risk factor for the disease
Confounding	The distortion or masking of an association between an exposure and outcome by the presence of a third variable

Related Principles
Relative risk (Measures of frequency and association)
Causation (Causality)
Case-control, retrospective studies (Observational studies)
Models for causation (Causality)

References
Caan, B.J., and Goldhaber, M.K. 1989. Caffeinated beverages and low birthweight: a case-control study. Am. J. Pub. Health 79: 1299-1300.
Dales, L.G., and Ury, H.K. 1978. An improper use of statistical significance testing in studying variables. Int. J. of Epidemiol. 7: 373-375.
Hogue, C.J. 1981. Coffee in pregnancy. Lancet 1: 554.

MacMahon, B., Yen, S., Trichopoulos, D., et al. 1981. Coffee and cancer of the pancreas. N. Engl. J. Med. 304:630-633.

McDonald, A.D., Armstrong, B.G., and Sloan, M. 1992. Cigarette, alcohol, and coffee consumption and prematurity. Am. J. Pub. Health 82:87-90.

Miettinen, O. 1974. Confounding and effect-modification. Am. J. of Epidemiol. 100:350-353.

Miettinen, O.S. 1976. Stratification by a multivariate confounder score. Am. J of Epidemiol. 104:609-620.

Miettinen, O., and Cook, E.F. 1981. Confounding: essence and definition. Am. J. of Epidemiol. 114: 593-603.

Olsen, J., Overvad, K., and Frische, G. 1991. Coffee consumption, birthweight, and reproductive failures. Epidemiol. 2:370-374.

Peacock, J.L., Bland, J.M., and Anderson, H.R. 1991. Effects on birthweight of alcohol and caffeine consumption in smoking women. J. Epidemiol. Community Health 45:159-163.

Rothman, K.J. 1975. A pictorial representation of confounding in epidemiological studies. J. of Chronic Disease. 32: 101-108.

Susser, D. 1973. Causal thinking in the health sciences. Concepts and strategies in epidemiology. Oxford University Press, New York.

Weinberg, C.R. 1993. Toward a clearer definition of confounding. Am. J. of Epidemiol. 137: 1-8.

Wold, H. 1956. Causal inference from observational data (with discussion). J. of the Royal Statistical Society, Series A. 119: 28-61.

Bias and Error: Study Questions

1. Which forms of bias are more relevant to case-control studies?
2. Which biases are more relevant to cohort studies?
3. Explain the differences between random and nonrandom bias.
4. Give an example of a study involving a particular exposure and disease that would be complicated because of confounding. What is the confounder? How would you control the confounding?
5. What are the criteria to establish when determining the presence of confounding? What is one way to prove the presence of confounding?
6. What is the difference between bias and error?
7. What is the specific situation that must be present in all of the types of selection bias?
8. Give another example of a disease that would be affected by lead-time bias.
9. Explain the differences between nondifferential and differential misclassification.
10. Why does differential misclassification have more of an effect on the validity of a study?

CHAPTER 7

Causality

One assumption that epidemiologists must be careful not to make is that an association between an exposure and disease proves that an exposure causes the disease. In fact, epidemiologists are so careful about this assumption that they are often hesitant to make a strong statement, such as factor x causes disease y. Instead, a statement of **Causation** is often phrased, "may cause," "may influence," "could increase," or is "strongly associated." One reason for the hesitancy is that observational studies do not often allow direct determination of a cause and effect. Also the study of disease is complex. Many factors may cause a disease and these factors may be interrelated; conversely, one factor may cause several diseases. Rarely is there a one-to-one relationship. **Models for Causation** have been developed over the years in an attempt to explain the causation of disease and the interrelationships of factors causing disease, such as the host, agent of disease, environment, and genetic variables.

Obviously, to make a decision about causation, there must be an association between the exposure and disease. Although there are several types of associations, there must be a statistically significant direct association. The biggest criterion for causation is that a change in exposure brings about a change in the outcome or disease.

Although a direct association is important, the final decision is made after careful analyses of the data. Several accepted criteria are used by epidemiologists to make a decision regarding causality. Since there are disagreements about which criteria are the most important, all are considered, and no criterion stands alone in making the decision about causality.

Historically, the use of criteria to determine causality began with Koch's postulates. In 1882 Robert Koch discovered the organism that causes tuberculosis. In his search, along with other scientists, to find the causes and treatments for the multiple infectious diseases resulting in deaths during the 19th century, Koch developed criteria for determining the organism that causes an infectious disease. His objective criteria were one of the first attempts to establish requirements for determining causation. His postulates were: (1) an organism must be found in all diseased cases; (2) the organism must be isolated from diseased patients and grown in culture; (3) the organism, when retrieved from the pure culture, must cause the same disease in inoculated animals; and (4) the organism must then be able to be isolated from the diseased animals and grown on pure culture. Koch's postulates remain a classic example of determining the cause of an infectious disease by a microorganism.

In this chapter the criteria used by epidemiologists to make a decision about causality are discussed. Each criterion is treated as a separate principle and is presented in recognized order of importance. They are **Strength of Association, Consistency of Effect, Biologic Plausibility, Dose-Response, Temporal Sequence, and Specificity of Effect.** The same disease example is used for each criterion to give this chapter continuity. It is a familiar example used in other texts because the example demonstrates most of the criteria used to establish causality. In most cases of determining causality, only a few of the criteria are met, and a decision has to be made as to whether there is enough evidence for causality. The material used for the examples for the criteria is based on a report from an advisory committee that was formed in 1960 to advise the Surgeon General about the risk of cigarette smoking and lung cancer. A panel of experts from various medical fields studied the evidence and gave their recommendation to the Surgeon General.

List of Principles

Causation An association is simply a relationship between two variables. The presence of an association does not mean that the relationship is causal. Causation is the ability of a factor to produce an effect or change in the disease. Causality is that relationship between the cause and effect.

Models for Causation Determining the cause of disease is a complex, interrelated process. It is rare to find one variable that will directly cause one disease. Models or theories of causation have been developed to help the understanding and study of the disease process.

Strength of Association A disease is rarely caused by one factor. Determining how important a specific factor is in the development of a disease may be difficult. Measuring the strength of association between a specific factor and the disease allows its importance to be quantified. The stronger the association, the more likely the factor is to be a cause of the disease.

Consistency of Effect   In observational studies it is important to validate the results with other studies. Since controlled experiments are not possible, replications of the study in other populations and by different study designs can validate original conclusions.

Biologic Plausibility   A statistically significant association is useless for proving causation unless the mechanisms by which the associated risk factor causes the disease make biologic or etiologic sense.

Dose-Response   Dose-response is related to the strength of association. As the dose increases, the more likely the risk of disease and the stronger the association. Duration of exposure can also be considered as dose. The longer an individual is exposed, the more likelihood there is for the individual to develop disease.

Temporal Sequence   Causation is not possible without the cause occurring before the effect. The time period between the exposure and disease must make biologic sense, especially if the disease is cancer. The temporal sequence can only be determined with prospective studies.

Specificity of Effect   The specificity of an effect is often difficult to demonstrate because most diseases are caused by multiple factors. If a factor causes a specific disease, this is good evidence of causality. A strong association of an effect, among other effects, in causing a particular disease can also be evidence of specificity.

Causation

An association is simply a relationship between two variables. The presence of an association does not mean that the relationship is causal. Causation is the ability of a factor to produce an effect or change in the disease. Causality is that relationship between the cause and effect.

Explanation

The first step in establishing causation is to determine if there is an association between two variables. An indirect or direct association can be determined statistically between two variables. A direct statistical association is the only type of association that could qualify as a causal relationship. When there is a true causal relationship, a change in the one variable causes a change in the other variable. An indirect association can be demonstrated statistically, but it is usually due to the presence of another variable that is common to the other two variables. In such case, a change in the risk factor does not cause a change in the disease *unless* the change affects the other variable that is common to both. The statistical association is determined by the testing of hypotheses, the p-values, and confidence intervals. If the association is statistically significant, it is less likely to be due to chance and is probably a true association.

A spurious, or artifactual association, is important to avoid. A spurious association is an association that shows up statistically but does not really exist. This usually occurs because of chance or a biased, incorrect observation. The act of accepting that association is also called a type I error. A type I error occurs when the null hypothesis is rejected and there really is no difference. A biased observation may be caused by a non-blinded interviewer asking leading questions to respondents and therefore receiving biased answers. A spurious association can also occur in case-control studies when the selection of the control group is biased in such a way that the controls are different from the cases in a factor that influences the disease being studied.

The magnitude of the association between a risk factor and a disease can also help in the evaluation of whether the association is true or artifactual. One statistical measure of the magnitude of the association is the correlation coefficient. Correlation coefficients can measure the strength or degree of the association, as well as the direction of the association. Correlational coefficients are often calculated by linear regression; therefore they evaluate the linear relationship of the two variables. In other words, an increase in one variable (the risk factor) can cause a linear increase or decrease in the other variable (disease). The numerical value, 0 to 1, reflects the degree of association; that is, as the variable or exposure changes, so does the outcome or disease. If there is no linear association, the correlation coefficient is 0. If there is a strong linear association, then the coefficient is 1. A value of 0.2 or less may mean a weak association and a value of 0.7 or higher may mean a strong association. The sign of the numerical value tells the direction of the relationship. A positive sign means that as the variable increases, the outcome also increases. A negative sign means that as the variable increases, the outcome decreases, but they are still associated.

Causal relationships may be direct or indirect and may involve one factor producing a disease or numerous factors producing a disease. Rarely, does just one factor produce a disease. More frequently, the process is much more complex. For example, one agent may cause several diseases. The human immunodeficiency virus (HIV) causes a number of syndromes affecting various organ systems that are considered part of the acquired immunodeficiency disease syndrome (AIDS). Likewise, one disease may be caused by various factors. Coronary heart disease can be caused by factors such as high cholesterol, genetic predisposition, stress, high alcohol intake, hypertension, and cigarette smoking. These factors may work separately, they may work together, or they may be one step in a chain of events leading to coronary heart disease. For example, a genetic predisposition to hypertension in combination with obesity may lead to hypertension. Hypertension, in turn, if not controlled, may cause coronary heart disease.

Example

A study of foresters and accountants shows that accountants have a higher risk of coronary heart disease. The assumption is that accounting is the occupation that causes the higher risk. However, a change in jobs may or may not affect the risk of coronary heart disease. It is not the job, but rather the influences of diet, family history, and exercise, that determine the risk of coronary heart disease. Foresters spend most of their time outside and generally stay in excellent physical shape. Accountants are in sedentary jobs and unless they exercise outside the job, get much less exercise. The more exercise and physical activity, the less the risk of coronary heart disease.

TERMS

Association	Relationship between two variables
Causation	The ability of one variable, the cause, to produce a change in another variable, the effect
Causality	The relationship between cause and effect
Cause	A variable that brings about a change or an effect
Correlation	How variables change with each other
Correlation Coefficient	A measurement of the strength and direction of association of variables
Spurious Association	An artifactual association that is not actually true

Related Principles

Level of significance, type I, type II error (Basic epidemiologic methodology)

Models for causation

Strength of association

Selection bias (Bias and error)

Information bias (Bias and error)

Blinding (Basic epidemiologic methodology)

References

Huck, S.W., Cormier, W.H., and Bounds, W.G. 1974. Reading statistics and research. Harper and Row, New York.

Kleinbaum, D.G., and Kupper, L.L. 1978. Applied regression analysis and other multivariable methods. Duxbury Press. North Scituate, Massachusetts.

Ott, L. 1984. An introduction to statistical methods and data analysis. Second Edition. PWS Publishers, Duxbury Press. Boston, Massachusetts.

Rothman, K.J. 1982. Causation and causal inference. In Schottenfield, D., and Fraumeni, J.F.(eds.). Cancer epidemiology and prevention. W.B. Saunders. Philadelphia, Pennsylvania.

Rothman, K.J. 1988. Causal inference. Epidemiology Resources. Chestnut Hill, Massachusetts.

Susser, M. 1973. Causal thinking in the health sciences. Oxford University Press, New York.

Weiss, N.S., and Liff, J.M. 1983. Accounting for the multicausal nature of disease in the design and analysis of epidemiologic studies. Am. J. Epidemiol. 117:14-18.

Models for Causation

Determining the cause of disease is a complex, interrelated process. It is rare to find one variable that will directly cause one disease. Models or theories of causation have been developed to help the understanding and study of the disease process.

Explanation

Epidemiology is the scientific inquiry into the causation of disease. In other words, it is the search for the risk factors that cause the effect or disease. In this search, various theories have evolved in an attempt to explain the interaction of risk factors and their effect on disease. Although the models differ in their emphasis of importance of the various components, all of them have the same components: host, agent, and environment. The models can be used for infectious and chronic diseases.

Earlier theories divided causation simply into intrinsic or host factors, such as immunity, genetics, personality, and extrinsic or environmental factors, such as biology, sociology, and culture. Ecologic models combined the biologic, social, and cultural environments together. An older common theory of causation, the epidemiologic triangle (Fig. 7-1 in Example 1), was one of the first models to make the agent an equal component of causation along with the host and environment. This triangle implies that all components are equally important in disease causation and that a change in any one of them would change the frequency of disease. Although this model is still appropriate for infectious diseases, more complicated chronic diseases required more sophisticated models of causation. Three newer models are worth mentioning.

The web of causation is one of the most commonly used. It merely reflects the fact that there is a complex mixture or a "web" of factors that can cause disease. These factors include different host, environmental, and other factors that may be interrelated and can act in various ways to cause disease. This model conveys a large quantity of information about a complex disease process.

The wheel model (Fig. 7-2 in Example 2) also depicts multiple factors that may cause disease. However, the wheel model does separate the roles of the host, environmental influences, and genetic factors. This model places genetic factors in the core of the wheel and varies the size of the host and environmental components depending on their influence in the particular disease process.

Rothman has proposed a pie-shaped model called the causal pie that has factors causing disease represented by pieces of that pie. Rothman defines both necessary and sufficient causes. A necessary cause is a cause that must be present but might not be the cause of a disease to develop. A sufficient cause is one that always results in disease. The whole pie is the sufficient cause for disease. There may be one or more pies, or sufficient causes, for one disease. If the same piece of pie, or factor, is in several of the pies, then that particular factor is considered a necessary cause. For example, the organism, *Mycobacterium sp.*, is necessary to cause tuberculosis in people and animals but not every human or animal exposed to *Mycobacterium sp.* gets tuberculosis. Other factors, such as a person's immune system, affect whether a person gets tuberculosis. It is logical that no matter what model of causation is used in describing the cause of a disease, the more factors involved, the more complicated the model, and the more difficult the determination of all of the causes.

Models of causation are important not only for determining the cause of disease but also for the prevention and control of disease. Prevention and control of a disease sometimes can be accomplished by focusing on just several of the most important factors. The models help to focus on several factors and their interrelationships and to speculate on how the disease may be affected by control of the factors.

Examples

1. Epidemiologic triangle:

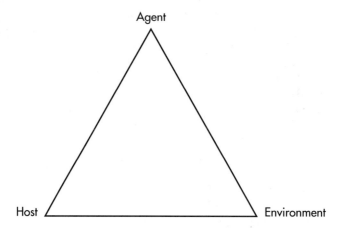

Fig. 7-1   Epidemiologic triangle model of causation. (From CDC, Epidemiology Program Office, Public Health Practice Program Office, DHHS. 1992. Principles of epidemiology, Second edition. Self-study course 3030-G.)

2. Wheel of causation:

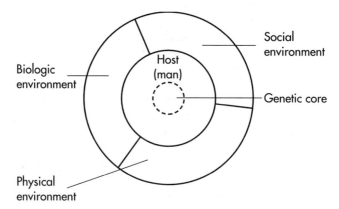

Fig. 7-2   Wheel model of causation. (From Mausner, J.S., and Kramer, S. 1985. Mausner and Bahn, Epidemiology: an introductory text. W.B. Saunders, Philadelphia, Pennsylvania.)

TERMS

Agent	A factor necessary but not a sufficient cause of disease
Causation	The act of causing an effect
Necessary Cause	A factor that has to be present, but does not necessarily cause a disease to develop
Sufficient Cause	This factor always causes disease

Related Principles
Causation
Prevention and control (Overview)
Modes of transmission (Epidemiologic concepts of disease)

References
Evans, A.S. 1978. Causation and disease: a chronologic journey. Am. J. of Epidemiol. 108: 249-258.
Hill, A.B. 1965. The environment and disease: association or causation? Proceedings of the Royal Society of Medicine. 58:295-300.
MacMahon, B., and Pugh, T.F. 1970. Epidemiologic principles and methods. Little, Brown, and Company. Boston, Massachusetts.
Mausner, J.S., and Kramer, S. 1985. Mausner and Bahn, Epidemiology: an introductory text. W.B. Saunders. Philadelphia, Pennsylvania.
Rothman, K.J. 1986. Modern epidemiology. Little, Brown, and Company, Boston, Massachusetts.
Susser, M. 1977. Judgment and causal inference: criteria in epidemiologic studies. Am. J. Epidemiol. 105:1-15.
Susser, M. 1973. Causal thinking in the health sciences. Oxford University Press, New York.

Strength of Association

A disease is rarely caused by one factor. Determining how important a specific factor is in the development of a disease may be difficult. Measuring the strength of association between a specific factor and the disease allows its importance to be quantified. The stronger the association, the more likely the factor is to be a cause of the disease.

Explanation

Usually there are several causes of a disease, and it is difficult to establish a one-to-one relationship between one cause and one disease. Determining the strength of the association is one of the major criteria in determining the cause of a disease. Depending on the type of study, it may be fairly easy to get a numerical value to express the strength of the association. The stronger the association, the more likely the relationship is causal. If the data are available, the strength of association can be measured by the relative risk, odds ratio, or a correlation coefficient. Therefore prospective and retrospective studies can estimate the strength of the association between a risk factor and a disease. The estimates of the strength help determine the relative importance of this factor in causing the disease.

There is no magic number that says the association is strong enough to be a cause; however, it is logical that the larger the relative risk, the more likely that the factor is the cause of the disease. Weak associations are more likely to be caused by error or chance.

Attributable risk can also give a good estimate of the strength of the association because it calculates directly how much of the disease in the population is due to the factor. As discussed in Chapter 3, the attributable risk measures the excess risk of disease in the exposed population compared to the nonexposed population.

Example (The first use of common smoking example.)

In 1960 the relationship of cigarette smoking and lung cancer was explored by an advisory committee to the Surgeon General. Three prospective studies (Doll and Hill, 1956; Hammond and Horn, 1958; and Dorn, 1958) showed strong statistical associations between cigarette smoking and lung cancer. The ratio of mortality rates of heavy smokers to nonsmokers was 20 to 1 in the studies of Hammond and Dorn and 40 to 1 in Doll's. In Doll's study the age-adjusted death rate (> 35 years of age) for lung cancer per year per 1000 men was 0.90 for smokers and 0.07 for nonsmokers, and the calculated relative risk for smokers compared to nonsmokers for dying of lung cancer was 12 per 1000.

TERMS

Strength of Association	How strong the association is between the factor of interest and the disease

Related Principles

Attributable risk (Measures of frequency and association)
Relative risk (Measures of frequency and association)
Odds ratio (Measures of frequency and association)
Causation
Prospective, cohort studies (Observational studies)
Case-control, retrospective studies (Observational studies)

References

Doll, R., and Hill, A.B. 1956. Lung cancer and other causes of death in relation to smoking. A second report on the mortality of British doctors. Br. Med. J. 2:1071-1081. (The first preliminary report was in 1950.)

Dorn, H.F. 1958. The mortality of smokers and non-smokers. Proc. Soc. Stat. Sect. Am. Stat. Assoc. 1:34.

Hammond, E.C., and Horn, D. 1958. Smoking and death rates: report on forty-four months of follow-up on 187,783 men. II: Death rates by cause. JAMA 166: 1294-1308.

Mausner, J.S., and Kramer, S. 1985. Mausner and Bahn, Epidemiology: an introductory text. W.B. Saunders. Philadelphia, Pennsylvania.

Roht, L.H., Selwyn B.J., Holguin, A.H., and Christensen, B.L. 1982. Principles of epidemiology: a self-teaching guide. Academic Press. Orlando, Florida.

U.S. Dept of HEW. 1964. Smoking and health: report of the advisory committee to the Surgeon General of the Public Health Service. USPHS Pub. No. 1103. U.S. Govt. Printing Office, Washington, D.C.

Consistency of Effect

In observational studies it is important to validate the results with other studies. Since controlled experiments are not possible, replications of the study in other populations and by different study designs can validate original conclusions.

Explanation

Since epidemiology is an inexact science, there is always some doubt about the results. If the same results are achieved in various types of studies, in different populations, and under different circumstances, epidemiologists are more confident of their results. For example, analyses can be done on several subgroups in the population, such as different age groups, to see if the same trend or effect occurs. Different studies, such as prospective or retrospective, can be done to see if the same results occur.

The evidence for causality is stronger when similar results are reached by various researchers with different types of studies; the same results are less likely to occur by chance. A new method of analysis, meta-analysis, has become popular in an attempt to quantify different studies investigating the same hypothesis. Meta-analysis evaluates similar types of studies looking at the same hypothesis and combines their results on the same statistical scale. This allows evaluation of the results to give an overall score. The use and methods of meta-analysis are still very controversial among epidemiologists.

Example

The advisory committee report to the Surgeon General stated the results of various prospective studies, laboratory experiments, and retrospective studies. Over 20 retrospective studies using different cases, various control groups, and measurements determined high relative risks for smokers versus nonsmokers. In all of the retrospective studies, male smokers had higher relative risks of lung cancer than male nonsmokers. The relative risks ranged from 4.6 to 34.1.

Laboratory studies have also found a significant risk for lung cancer caused by tobacco smoke in several different species of animals. Laboratory studies demonstrated that there were carcinogenic substances in tobacco smoke capable of producing cancer or cancerous changes. Tobacco tar and benzopyrene applied to the skin of mice and rabbits produced tumors. Cigarette smoke condensates injected subcutaneously in rats and aerosol applications to the lungs of mice, rats, hamsters, and primates produced cancerous lesions.

TERMS

Consistency	Showing steady conformity and continuity; regularity. Agreement of several with one another or with the whole

Related Principles
Biologic plausibility
Interdisciplinary nature (Overview)

References

Dickerson, K., and Berlin, J.A. 1992. Meta-analysis: state of the science. Epidemiologic Reviews 14:154-176.

Doll, R., and Hill, A.B. 1956. Lung cancer and other causes of death in relation to smoking. A second report on the mortality of British doctors. Br. Med. J. 2:1071-1081. (The first preliminary report was in 1950.)

Dorn, H.F. 1958. The mortality of smokers and non-smokers. Proc. Soc. Stat. Sect. Am. Stat. Assoc. 1:34.

Fleiss, J.L., and Gross, A.J. (eds.) 1991. Meta-analysis in epidemiology, with special reference to studies of the association between exposure to environmental tobacco smoke and lung cancer: a critique. J. Clin. Epidemiol. 44:127-139.

Hammond, E.C., and Horn, D. 1958. Smoking and death rates: report on forty-four months of follow-up on 187,783 men. II: Death rates by cause. JAMA 166: 1294-1308.

Mausner, J.S., and Kramer, S. 1985. Mausner and Bahn, Epidemiology: an introductory text. W.B. Saunders. Philadelphia, Pennsylvania.

U.S. Dept of HEW. 1964. Smoking and health: report of the advisory committee to the Surgeon General of the Public Health Service. USPHS Pub. No. 1103. U.S. Govt. Printing office, Washington, D.C.

Webster's New Collegiate Dictionary. 1974. G and C Merriam Co.. Springfield, Massachusetts.

Biologic Plausibility

A statistically significant association is useless for proving causation unless the mechanisms by which the associated risk factor causes the disease make biologic or etiologic sense.

Explanation

Once a possible causal relationship has been established, the mechanism by which the exposure causes disease must make biologic or etiologic sense. In other words, has there been animal or in vitro studies performed that show the pathogenesis of the disease? Even though the pathogenesis may not be completely understood, does the proposed mechanism make biologic sense? Is it consistent with existing knowledge? For example, does the exposure contain carcinogens? Is there histologic or pathologic evidence of carcinogenesis? Can the exposure result in contact with the organ system affected by disease? If the exposure is to an infectious organism, is there a gradient of severity of disease that correlates with the infectious level of the organism?

Example

Several types of laboratory studies showed that components of tobacco smoke were carcinogens to the skin, subcutaneous tissue, and lung tissue. In addition, the act of smoking brings these carcinogens in contact with delicate lung tissues. Pathologic studies of smokers and nonsmokers showed obvious epithelial changes in the lungs of smokers. Other pathologic studies were done on beagles, hamsters, and rats that were exposed through tracheostomy tubes or intratracheal exposure to tobacco smoke. These animals developed pulmonary tumors.

TERMS

Plausibility	Reasonable, believable

Related Principles
Consistency of effect

References

Doll, R., and Hill, A.B. 1956. Lung cancer and other causes of death in relation to smoking. A second report on the mortality of British doctors. Br. Med. J. 2:1071-1081. (The first preliminary report was in 1950.)

Dorn, H.F. 1958. The mortality of smokers and non-smokers. Proc. Soc. Stat. Sect. Am. Stat. Assoc. 1:34.

Hammond, E.C., and Horn, D. 1958. Smoking and death rates: report on forty-four months of follow-up on 187,783 men. II: Death rates by cause. JAMA 166: 1294-1308.

Mausner, J.S., and Kramer, S. 1985. Mausner and Bahn, Epidemiology: an introductory text. W.B. Saunders. Philadelphia, Pennsylvania.

U.S. Dept of HEW. 1964. Smoking and Health: Report of the advisory committee to the Surgeon General of the Public Health Service. USPHS Pub. No. 1103. U.S. Govt. Printing Office, Washington, D.C.

Dose-Response

Dose-response is related to the strength of association. As the dose increases, the more likely the risk of disease and the stronger the association. Duration of exposure can also be considered as dose. The longer an individual is exposed, the more likelihood there is for the individual to develop disease.

Explanation

This concept is similar to the strength of association. If higher doses cause larger responses, it demonstrates a direct effect between exposure and disease and, therefore causation. This is often difficult to demonstrate, but it can be shown for environmental exposures, toxins, and even infectious organisms. The dose-response can be shown by calculating the relative risk for subgroups of the population according to the magnitude of each subgroup's exposure. An example is to look at the effect of cholesterol level on the risk of heart disease. Compare a group of men with cholesterol levels of < 200, 201 to 300, and > 300. Men with cholesterol levels of > 300 have a much higher risk of heart disease than those with lower levels, and men with levels of < 200 have the lowest risk of heart disease. The duration of exposure can also be used as a measure of dose. In this case, the longer an individual is exposed, the more likely the risk of developing disease. For example, the longer an individual smokes, the higher the risk of developing lung cancer.

However, caution must be used when making the judgment of dose-response because dose-response does not necessarily mean cause and effect. There may be another reason for the apparent dose-response. For example, there were reports of a dose-response between the number of cups of coffee that were drunk and the likelihood of the development of lung cancer. These reports were incorrect. After further examination, these studies also had shown that cigarette smokers often smoked when they drank coffee and that they were heavy coffee drinkers. It was not the coffee drinking but rather the cigarette smoking that was causing the lung cancer.

Example
The three prospective studies referred to earlier in the chapter show a dose-response. The mortality rates increased with the number of cigarettes smoked per day.

MORTALITY RATES

Dose	Doll Study	Hammond Study	Dorn Study
< 10 cig/day	4.4	5.8	5.2
10-20 cig/day	10.8	7.3	9.4
> 40 cig/day	43.7	21.7	23.3

TERMS

Dose-Response   A change in the duration or amount of exposure is associated with change in the risk of disease

Related Principles
Strength of association

References
Doll, R., and Hill, A.B. 1956. Lung cancer and other causes of death in relation to smoking. A second report on the mortality of British doctors. Br. Med. J. 2:1071-1081. (The first preliminary report was in 1950.)

Dorn, H.F. 1958. The mortality of smokers and non-smokers. Proc. Soc. Stat. Sect. Am. Stat. Assoc. 1:34.

Hammond, E.C., and Horn, D. 1958. Smoking and death rates: report on forty-four months of follow-up on 187,783 men. II: Death rates by cause. JAMA 166: 1294-1308.

Mausner, J.S., and Kramer, S. 1985. Mausner and Bahn, Epidemiology: an introductory text. W.B. Saunders. Philadelphia, Pennsylvania.

U.S. Dept of HEW. 1964. Smoking and health: report of the advisory committee to the Surgeon General of the Public Health Service. USPHS Pub. No. 1103. U.S. Govt. Printing Office, Washington, D.C.

Temporal Sequence

Causation is not possible without the cause occurring before the effect. The time period between the exposure and disease must make biologic sense, especially if the disease is cancer. The temporal sequence can only be determined with prospective studies.

Explanation

Obviously, the cause must come before the effect, and the time interval from exposure to disease must make biologic sense. For example, cancer takes time to develop. It is unlikely for a person to be exposed to a suspected risk factor, develop cancer 2 weeks later, and the risk factor considered a cause of that cancer. Animal studies are helpful in studying the causes of cancer because animals have much shorter life spans than humans and develop cancer much more quickly than humans. These studies provide the opportunity to study the effects of carcinogens much more quickly. The temporal sequence is more easily determined with environmental or occupational exposures or in acute outbreaks of disease than with chronic diseases.

Temporal trends cannot be determined by cross-sectional or retrospective studies. The only way to determine temporal trends is through prospective studies. There must be a determination of the exposure occurring before the disease. Prospective studies define the exposure in the beginning and follow the individuals until they develop the disease. The temporal sequence is defined and incidence rates are measured. If a temporal sequence between exposure and disease can be established, then there is further evidence of causality.

Example

Studies have shown that by quitting smoking the damaged lung tissue over time returns to normal. The fact that the lung tissue becomes healthy again may decrease the chances of developing lung cancer compared to lung tissue exposed to smoking. The longer the person has stopped smoking, the less likely the risk of lung cancer compared to when smoking. In Hammonds and Horns' study, the lung cancer incidence decreased in proportion to the amount of time the individuals had stopped smoking.

MORTALITY RATE

	< 1 pack/day	> 1 pack/day
Still smoke	57.6	157.1
Stopped < 1 yr	56.1	198
Stopped 1-10 yr	35.5	77.6
Stopped > 10 yr	8.3	60.5

TERMS

Temporal	Passage in time

Related Principles
Cross-sectional, survey studies (Observational studies)
Case-control, retrospective studies (Observational studies)
Prospective, cohort studies (Observational studies)
Person, place, and time (Epidemiologic concepts of disease)
Incidence, prevalence (Measures of frequency and association)

References
Doll, R., and Hill, A.B. 1956. Lung cancer and other causes of death in relation to smoking. A second report on the mortality of British doctors. Br. Med. J. 2:1071-1081. (The first preliminary report was in 1950.)

Dorn, H.F. 1958. The mortality of smokers and non-smokers. Proc. Soc. Stat. Sect. Am. Stat. Assoc. 1:34.

Hammond, E.C., and Horn, D. 1958. Smoking and death rates: report on forty-four months of follow-up on 187,783 men. II: Death rates by cause. JAMA 166: 1294-1308.

Mausner, J.S., and Kramer, S. 1985. Mausner and Bahn, Epidemiology: an introductory text. W.B. Saunders. Philadelphia, Pennsylvania.

U.S. Dept of HEW. 1964. Smoking and health: report of the advisory committee to the Surgeon General of the Public Health Service. USPHS Pub. No. 1103. U.S. Govt. Printing Office, Washington, D.C.

Specificity of Effect

The specificity of an effect is often difficult to demonstrate because most diseases are caused by multiple factors. If a factor causes a specific disease, this is good evidence of causality. A strong association of an effect, among other effects, in causing a particular disease can also be evidence of specificity.

Explanation

Specificity means that a cause leads to one effect rather than multiple effects. It is rare to find a one-to-one relationship. The taking of diethylstilbestrol (DES) by pregnant women and the occurrence of vaginal carcinoma in their daughters is one example of a specific effect. Most variables can cause several diseases just as most diseases are caused by multiple factors. This criterion cannot be independent of the strength of association. The stronger the degree of association for one disease, compared to other diseases, and the factor of interest, the more specific the relationship. Attributable risk and relative risk can be a measure of specificity. Attributable risk estimates the excess risk of disease in a population for a specific exposure. For example, lung cancer mortality is much higher among smokers than any other causes of death, such as bladder cancer, that also might be related to smoking. This criterion is very difficult to show but if it is present, it is very good evidence of causality. If specificity cannot be demonstrated, it does not mean that there is not causation.

Example

This is the most controversial criterion for showing causality for cigarette smoking and lung cancer. Lung cancer is not the only disease caused by smoking; smoking is also linked with coronary heart disease and other respiratory diseases. Tobacco smoke is made up of a complex mixture of benzopyrene, tar, nicotine, and other substances that are considered carcinogenic. They may work in different ways on different tissues. The strongest suggestion of specificity is the strength of association compared to the other disease. The risk of smokers for lung cancer is 10 times that of nonsmokers. By comparison, the risk of smokers for coronary heart disease is 1.7 times that of nonsmokers.

TERMS

Specificity	The development of a certain disease being unique to a particular exposure

Related Principles
Strength of association
Dose-response
Attributable risk (Measures of frequency and association)
Relative risk (Measures of frequency and association)

References
Doll, R., and Hill, A.B. 1956. Lung cancer and other causes of death in relation to smoking. A second report on the mortality of British doctors. Br. Med. J. 2:1071-1081. (The first preliminary report was in 1950.)

Dorn, H.F. 1958. The mortality of smokers and non-smokers. Proc. Soc. Stat. Sect. Am. Stat. Assoc. 1:34.

Hammond, E.C., and Horn, D. 1958. Smoking and death rates: report on forty-four months of follow-up on 187,783 men. II: Death rates by cause. JAMA 166: 1294-1308.

Mausner, J.S., and Kramer, S. 1985. Mausner and Bahn, Epidemiology: an introductory text. W.B. Saunders. Philadelphia, Pennsylvania.

U.S. Dept of HEW. 1964. Smoking and Health: Report of the advisory committee to the Surgeon General of the Public Health Service. USPHS Pub. No. 1103. U.S. Govt. Printing Office, Washington, D.C.

Causality: Study Questions

1. Give examples of an indirect noncausal relationship, an indirect *causal* relationship, and a direct causal relationship. Explain the differences.
2. Give at least two examples of situations that might lead to a spurious association.
3. What is the meaning of a correlation coefficient of 0.78 between the miles of walking done every day and your blood pressure? What if the correlation coefficient was −0.34?
4. For each model for causation, the epidemiologic triangle, the wheel, the web, and Rothman's sufficient causal pie, choose a disease that would be appropriately explained by the model selected.
5. Explain the difference between necessary and sufficient cause and give examples of each.
6. Explain the difference between causation and causality.
7. List each criterion that is used for determining causality and explain its relative importance in the decision process.
8. Why does the fact that most diseases are not caused by a single factor cause problems in determining causality?
9. Why are the relative risk and attributable risk used to determine the strength of an association between variables? What do they tell you? Is this criterion related to dose-response?
10. Give another current example of a risk factor and disease causality that has been established by the results of different study designs and studies in different populations.
11. What is meant by biologic plausibility? Give an example.
12. Give a current example of a dose-response effect between an exposure and disease. What is the strength of this association when compared to other factors that might cause the same disease?
13. What types of study designs are useful to show a temporal sequence between an exposure and disease? Justify your answer.
14. Give an example of an exposure and disease that would demonstrate temporal sequence.
15. Give an example of a disease that is caused by a specific exposure or risk factor.
16. Explain Koch's postulates and give at least two examples of diseases that would fit under these postulates.

CHAPTER 8

Surveillance

Surveillance is the act of collecting data and using it to implement action. Surveillance provides important knowledge to epidemiologists about the occurrence of disease and events in a population, whether it is the frequency or distribution of a disease in a population or the use of a specific drug or device. Surveillance incorporates various methods of collecting data, analyzing and interpreting the data, and then initiating some form of action, either preventive or interventive. This action also includes the dissemination of information to health professionals and the public. In contrast, **Monitoring** is a less intensive form of surveillance. Monitoring programs collect information but take no action.

Surveillance is considered **Active or Passive** according to the data collected. If data are solicited from participating health agencies, the surveillance is active. If reports are submitted from health professionals or consumers voluntarily, then the surveillance is passive. Passive surveillance analyzes the data submitted by health professionals, which limits the information acquired, but the process is less costly and easier to maintain than active surveillance. Active surveillance requires the health agencies to solicit information. This process collects more detailed information but is more costly and requires much more effort than passive surveillance.

Screening programs, established by health agencies, are a form of surveillance for a specific disease to detect individuals in a population who are asymptomatic or have subclinical infections. The goal of a screening program is to detect subclinical individuals in order to initiate action. This may include either prevention of disease or control of the early stages of disease. Screening may also be used diagnostically to determine the frequency of a disease that was previously unknown in the population. Since it is difficult to conduct tests on a large population, it is important to focus on high-risk individuals or on a population that may have a high prevalence of the disease.

Screening programs involve a specific test for the disease. The **Sensitivity, Specificity, and Predictive Value** of this test are essential for the success of a screening program. The sensitivity and specificity determine the accuracy of the test; the accuracy is how well the test measures what it is supposed to measure. Sensitivity is the ability of the test to detect accurately an infected individual in the population. Specificity is the ability of the test to accurately detect an uninfected individual in the population. Sensitivity and specificity are inversely related to each other and are not affected by the prevalence of the disease in the population.

The predictive value is affected by the prevalence of a disease. The predictive value is the ability of the test to determine the absence or presence of the disease in a population. Obviously, the predictive value of a positive test is most important to a clinician who wants to detect disease in order to treat or control further disease.

List of Principles

Surveillance versus Monitoring	Monitoring is simply the observation and the analysis of routine measurements. The primary goal of monitoring is detection; it may detect a change or pattern in disease occurrence. Surveillance is a system that collects, analyzes, and interprets data on disease frequency and distribution in the population to initiate control measures or further investigative action.
Active versus Passive	Passive surveillance is an established system that collects reports that are sent by health professionals to health departments or disease registries. These systems are easy to maintain and are inexpensive. Active surveillance requires the health departments to go out and collect detailed information on a specific disease or problem. This surveillance is money- and labor-intensive but collects much more detailed data.
Screening	Screening is the process of using a test or diagnostic method to detect asymptomatic or subclinical individuals who appear healthy for the purposes of control or prevention of the disease. Screening is most effective in a high-risk population that has a fairly high prevalence of the disease.

Sensitivity	The sensitivity of a test is the number of diseased individuals in a population who actually test positive on that test. It is the probability of correctly identifying a diseased individual by a specific test.
Specificity	The specificity of a test is the ability, by way of a negative result to identify the number of healthy individuals. It is the probability of correctly identifying a healthy individual by a specific test. Specificity is inversely related to sensitivity.
Predictive Value	The predictive value of a specific test is the ability to predict the absence or presence of a disease. The predictive value is affected by the prevalence of the disease in the population being tested. The higher the prevalence, the better the predictive value. The predictive value of a positive test is the most important clinically to health professionals.

Surveillance versus Monitoring

Monitoring is simply the observation and the analysis of routine measurements. The primary goal of monitoring is detection; it may detect a change or pattern in disease occurrence. Surveillance is a system that collects, analyzes, and interprets data on disease frequency and distribution in the population to initiate control measures or further investigative action.

Explanation

Monitoring and surveillance are often used interchangeably because they are similar, but they have different meanings and goals. Monitoring is basically an observation and collection process. It is important for increasing knowledge about the disease or the population. Monitoring involves the observation and analysis of a disease or events to accomplish the goal of detecting changes in the frequency or distribution in the population. It involves the collection of complete information for assessment but usually determines the occurrence of an event or a disease less rapidly than a surveillance program.

Surveillance, on the other hand, is more active in the analysis, interpretation, and action on the results of the data collected. It is a systematic approach of collecting, analyzing, and interpreting data with the goal to initiate control measures or further investigative methods.

Surveillance can include any aspect relevant to the control of disease. It is important to interpret the data quickly to initiate further action; therefore the process attempts to determine as early as possible the occurrence and distribution of a disease or an event in a population. The information collected is then disseminated to health professionals or to the public.

Surveillance can be initiated to test a specific hypothesis, to survey a general or specific population, to survey disease indicators such as the animal population or reservoirs or vectors of disease, or to survey drug and biologic utilization of the population. During the planning and in the evaluating of a surveillance system, there are several issues to keep in mind: the importance of the health event; the objectives (including the case definition); the usefulness, the flexibility, and the simplicity of the system; the representativeness, the timeliness, and the accuracy and quickness of detection of new cases or epidemics.

Sources of data are important for the surveillance process. The most common sources of data are mortality records, or death certificates, morbidity reporting or reportable diseases required by law, the reporting of epidemics and field investigations, laboratory investigations, and surveys. Each source has advantages and disadvantages when used for surveillance purposes. Death certificates are a good source because a denominator or population at risk can be calculated with the census data. In addition, death certificates are fairly standardized, easy to obtain, and include other basic demographic information such as age, gender, race, and occupation. Since 1979 the National Center for Health Statistics (NCHS) has maintained a National Death Index that is used by researchers to obtain death certificate information for research purposes. Mortality records provide the opportunity to look at trends over person, place, and time, and can be an indicator of certain disease frequencies in the population. Two disadvantages of death certificates are the inconsistent coding of diagnoses by different professionals and the fact that highly fatal diseases are more likely to be represented. Also, death certificates request coding of primary and secondary causes of death. The interpretation, and therefore the listing of primary versus secondary causes, may differ among individuals filling out the certificates. This difference in interpretation and listing can influence the measurement of a particular disease. The primary cause of death, for example, may be listed for an individual as pulmonary edema and the secondary cause as coronary heart disease. When in actuality, coronary heart disease is the primary disease that causes the pulmonary edema. For the study of occupational diseases, death certificates provide both a source of the mortality and the occupation of individuals. Mortality ratios can be calculated and compared for each occupational group. Sometimes more information can be collected from the listed employers.

Other surveillance systems use birth certificates; congenital defect registries maintained by Centers for Disease Control and Prevention (CDC); different periodic surveys done in the United States by the National Center for Health Statistics; the Surveillance, Epidemiology and End Results Program (SEER) maintained by the National Cancer Institute, which has 11 population-based cancer registries; the reportable disease system (CDC); and the *Morbidity, Mortality, Weekly Report* (MMWR) that CDC publishes.

Surveillance can involve the monitoring of individuals in a hospital setting or the monitoring of health events in a population. Hospitals have infection control programs for the surveillance of infections caused from being in the hospital. These surveillance programs look for infectious disease cases, perform data analysis, and then initiate some type of control program. Most of these surveillance programs include surveillance of laboratory records, medical charts, and active surveillance of high-risk areas, such as pediatrics or the intensive-care unit for new infectious cases. Rates of infection can be calculated by surgical procedure, by ward or hospital wing, and by service (medical, surgical).

Each surveillance program must be planned to meet a particular objective. For infectious disease surveillance, the objectives are to identify newly diagnosed cases and high-risk groups, to understand the mode of transmission, and to control or eliminate disease transmission. Surveillance can collect baseline incidence data to detect the occurrence of an epidemic. Seasonal, temporal, geographic, and subgroup patterns are important for understanding the mode of transmission and for determining ways in which to control the disease. Seasonal and temporal trends can give information about times in which control programs should be implemented. Geographic and subgroup patterns help epidemiologists focus control programs in the most effective areas.

The pervasive problems that occur with any surveillance system are underreporting, lack of representativeness, inconsistency in definition, and the lag time between the occurrence of an event and the actual reporting. Most surveillance systems consist of events that are underreported unless there is aggressive, active solicitation of reports of a particular disease or event. Normally medical professionals do not report a disease or an event unless it is serious or of specific interest. This kind of reporting can lead to reports in a system from those most interested and may not be representative of the general population. Reporting from various sources usually has inherent differences in diagnosis or definition of a disease. Finally, in any surveillance system there is a period of time that passes between the event and the time that it gets reported.

Examples

1. **Monitoring System:**

    Dairy producers and veterinarians usually initiate a herd health program to monitor the health of the producer's dairy cow population. This program is focused at a herd or population level but also ensures individual cow health. The program includes monitoring diet intake, milk production levels, vaccination status, reproductive history, and the number and type of infections and antibiotic use.

2. **Surveillance System:**

    a. More than 30 states maintain a state cancer registry. The National Cancer Institute also maintains a SEER system (Surveillance, Epidemiology, End Results) system in over 11 states. This system identifies patients diagnosed with cancer within those 11 states, by state or region, and collects demographic data, the type, location, and treatment of the cancer.

    b. The Food and Drug Administration's (FDA's) Center for Drug Evaluation and Research, Center for Devices and Radiologic Health, Center for Veterinary Medicine, and Center for Biologic Evaluation and Research maintain postmarketing surveillance systems. These systems collect adverse event reports on biologics, veterinary and human drugs, and devices that occur in marketed products to detect possible safety problems. These adverse events are required to be reported by the manufacturer but are also reported by health professionals, medical facilities, and consumers.

TERMS

Monitoring	Collection and analysis of routine data for the detection of changes in disease frequency or distribution in a population
Nosocomial	Infection obtained because of being in a hospital; pertaining to the hospital setting
Surveillance	The systematic collection, analysis, and interpretation of data about the frequency and distribution of disease for the purposes of initiating control measures or further investigative procedures. It includes the dissemination of the information to health professionals and the community

Related Principles

Person, place, and time (Epidemiologic concepts of disease)
Active versus passive
Case definition (Epidemiologic concepts of disease)
Prevention and control (Overview)
Population medicine (Overview)

References

Brachman, P.S. 1982. Surveillance in bacterial infections of humans.
    Evans, A.S, and Feldman, H.L. (eds.). Plenum Press, New York.
CDC. 1990. Case definitions for public health surveillance. MMWR. 39:
    (RR-13) 1-43.
CDC. 1988. Guidelines for evaluating surveillance systems. MMWR. 37:
    (S-5) 1-18.
Evans, A.S. 1982. Surveillance and seroepidemiology in viral infections
    of humans. Plenum Press, New York.
Frazier, T.M., and Wegman, D.H. 1979. Exploring the use of death cer-
    tificates as a component of an occupational disease surveillance sys-
    tem. Am. J. Pub. Health 69: 718-720.
Langmuir, A.D. 1976. William Farr: founder of modern concepts of sur-
    veillance. Int. J. Epidemiol. 5: 13-18.
Langmuir, A.D. 1971. Evolution of the concept of surveillance in the
    United States. Proc. Roy. Soc. Med. 64:681-688.
Langmuir, A.D. 1963. The surveillance of communicable diseases of
    national importance. New. Engl. J. Med. 268: 182-192.
Raska, K. 1983. Epidemiologic surveillance in the control of infectious
    diseases. Rev. Infect. Dis. 5: 1112-1117.
Raska, K. 1966. National and international surveillance of communica-
    ble diseases. WHO Chron. 20: 313-321.
Thacker, S.B., Berkelman, R.L. 1988. Public health surveillance in the
    U.S.. Epidemiol. Rev. 10:164-190.
Thacker, S.B., Choi, K., Brachman, P.S. 1983. The surveillance of infec-
    tious disease. JAMA. 249: 1181-1185.
WHO. 1968. The surveillance of communicable disease. WHO Chroni-
    cle 22:439-444.

Active versus Passive

Passive surveillance is an established system that collects reports that are sent by health professionals to health departments or disease registries. These systems are easy to maintain and are inexpensive. Active surveillance requires the health departments to go out and collect detailed information on a specific disease or problem. This surveillance is money- and labor-intensive but collects much more detailed data.

Explanation

Passive surveillance collects information that is entered into an organized system. The information is sent by health professionals to the health departments, usually in response to rules or regulations. In other words, passive surveillance is initiated by the healthcare provider or even the consumer and does not involve active solicitation of data by health departments or agencies. Examples of passive surveillance systems are the state-reportable diseases, mandatory reporting of adverse drug or device reactions to the FDA, and cancer registries. Passive surveillance systems require little effort, are easy to maintain, and can offer basic information. Such basic data can be used to guide further investigations and to look for "signals" of potential increases in cases or problems.

There are, however, several disadvantages with a passive system. Underreporting is a major problem because there is no incentive to report other than an interest on the part of the medical professional or consumer or a regulation that may or may not be enforced. In passive systems, there is often an overrepresentation of the most commonly occurring diseases, well-publicized diseases, or diseases of most interest to physicians. In the case of adverse reporting of drugs and device problems, it is logical to assume that the drugs and devices used most often are more likely to have reported problems. Another disadvantage of a passive system, especially when trying to make useful conclusions from the data, is the fact that there is rarely a denominator or a population at risk. Conclusions about the data are limited.

Active surveillance is a process of collecting data for a period of time on a selected disease process and sometimes in a limited geographic region. The reports are solicited by the health department from health professionals; they are initiated by local, state, or federal health officials. Active surveillance may be used when a new syndrome has been reported, an epidemic has occurred, a new mode of transmission is discovered, or when there is a new geographic region or season affected. This surveillance collects more detailed information than the passive system.

The advantages of active surveillance are that this intensive effort collects detailed and complete information more representative of the true incidence of the disease of interest than the passive system. It also increases the number of reported cases; some would not have been reported under passive surveillance. Because active surveillance requires health departments to reach out to medical professionals, this process helps promote better cooperation among professionals and the health department. For example, NCHS conducts several types of surveys for different time periods on various interest areas. The results are published in a regular publication, *Vital and Health Statistics.* The major disadvantages are that this type of surveillance requires more funding, effort, and labor because the burden of reporting is placed on the public health agency; therefore active surveillance can only be pursued on a limited basis. Active surveillance is used for targeted investigations on a specific season or a geographically-defined area for a disease that can be affected by consequent control programs.

Examples
1. **Active Surveillance Systems:**
   a. During the influenza season, the CDC uses four active systems to collect information on the incidence of influenza: laboratories, mortality reports, physician network, and state epidemiologists. These systems collect weekly information:
      1. Influenza isolates from 60 state, city, and university laboratories
      2. The number and proportion of influenza deaths, attributable to pneumonia per week, by age, from 121 city mortality reporting systems
      3. The number of patients seen weekly with flulike symptoms from a sentinel physician system that includes a network of 150 physicians
      4. The assessment of each state epidemiologist about the level of influenza activity in their state.
   b. The NCHS conducts large surveys to look at a wide variety of health-related topics. For example, the National Health Interview Survey annually surveys a representative sample of about 130,000 people in 50,000 different households in the United States. Information is collected on demographic characteristics, illnesses, injuries, healthcare, and disabilities. The National Hospital Discharge Survey samples records of short-term and specialty hospitals for diagnoses and surgical procedures every couple of years. The National Ambulatory Medical Care Survey is conducted annually and requires about 3,000 sampled physicians to fill out patient record information about patients treated during a randomly selected week. The information includes diagnoses, treatments, and outcomes of the patients. The National Health and Nutrition Examination Surveys (NHANES I and II) were done from 1971 to 1975 and 1976 to 1980, respectively, to provide information on physical examinations and clinical and laboratory testing. At the same time, questionnaires were administered to a population of 20,000 individuals on nutrition, dental, skin, and eye problems, as well as on diabetes, kidney function, cardiovascular disease, and chronic arthritic conditions.

2. Passive Surveillance Systems:
   a. The council of state and territorial epidemiologists determines which diseases states should report to the CDC. This list is often revised every year. The CDC is also required to report the internationally quarantinable diseases to the World Health Organization; the diseases are plague, cholera, and yellow fever.
   b. The NCHS maintains the National Death Index, which contains the death certificates for the entire United States. A monthly national sample is taken and published in the *Vital and Health Statistics* every 3 months.

TERMS

Active Surveillance
A process initiated by health departments or agencies to collect reports on a specific disease for a limited period of time in a particular geographic area

Passive Surveillance
A surveillance system that maintains reports provided by health professionals to the health departments, agencies, or established disease registries

Related Principles
Surveillance versus monitoring
Cross-sectional, survey studies (Observational studies)

References
CDC, Epidemiology Program Office, Public Health Practice Program Office, DHHS. 1992. Principles of epidemiology, Second edition. Self-study course 3030-G.

Chorba, T.L., Berkelman, R.L., Safford, S.K., et al. 1989. The reportable disease. I: mandatory reporting of infectious diseases by clinicians. JAMA. 262:3018-3026.

Modesitt, S.K., Hulman, S., and Fleming, D. 1990. Evaluation of active versus passive AIDS surveillance in Oregon. Am. J. Public Health. 80: 463-464.

Nelson, C.R., and Stussman, B.J. 1994. Alcohol- and Drug-related visits to hospital emergency departments: 1992 National Hospital Ambulatory Medical Care Survey. Advance data from vital and health statistics, number 251. National Center for Health Statistics, Hyattsville, Maryland.

Reilly, M.J., Rosenman, K.D., Watt, F.C., et al. 1993. Silicosis surveillance: Michigan, New Jersey, Ohio, and Wisconsin, 1987-1990. In: CDC Surveillance Summaries, November 19, 1993. MMWR 42(No. SS-5): 23-28.

Screening

Screening is the process of using a test or diagnostic method to detect asymptomatic or subclinical individuals who appear healthy for the purposes of control or prevention of the disease. Screening is most effective in a high-risk population that has a fairly high prevalence of the disease.

Explanation

A screening program can be used for surveillance to get a better picture of the frequency of disease in the population. Primarily, screening is used to either detect individuals with the earliest symptoms of disease (subclinical) or used to identify individuals in a population who are infected but asymptomatic. In other words, screening allows the detection of people who appear to be healthy but really are diseased. The goal of a screening program is *not* to be diagnostic, but rather to identify individuals who are infected or who are in the early stages of disease so that the individuals can seek medical care and testing for final diagnosis. Early diagnosis can then lead to the initiation of preventive efforts. Screening programs are primarily aimed toward chronic diseases. These diseases have a longer natural history that allows an opportunity for prevention or early intervention to be successful.

There are different types of screening programs. Mass screening is rarely done because it is too expensive and labor-intensive to screen the entire population. Multiple or multiphasic screening can be done to increase the number of individuals detected. Multiphasic screening uses various screening tests at the same time to increase the number of positive individuals detected. Prescriptive screening is used for a disease where early detection can lead to better treatment or control of the disease if it is detected early. An example of prescriptive screening is the use of mammography to screen for early stages of breast cancer.

During implementation and in evaluation of screening programs, several issues need to be addressed: whether the disease is an important public health problem, whether there is a test that is able to detect asymptomatic disease, whether there are facilities for diagnosis and treatment, and whether there is an acceptable treatment. The test needs to be acceptable to the population and the cost reasonable relative to the benefits. A screening program is labor-intensive and costly; therefore it is only undertaken with diseases of public health importance in which intervention can be helpful. Because of the cost and the labor involved for screening programs, the programs are usually aimed at high-risk groups and in a population that has a high disease prevalence so that the most people who are infected can be detected. It is also important to realize that screening only detects prevalent cases. It is unknown whether these are new cases unless a repeat screening is done.

Obviously, the essential part of a screening program is the screening test; therefore it is important to evaluate the screening test. The validity of the test is how well it measures what it is supposed to be measuring. In other words, is the test result positive when the individual is diseased, and is the test result negative when the individual is healthy? The validity can be confirmed by comparing the screening test results with the results of the "gold standard" diagnostic tests. The reliability or precision of the test is the repeatability. When the test is repeated, are the same results obtained? The accuracy of the test is measured by whether the person is placed in the right category, diseased or nondiseased. The greater the validity, the greater the accuracy. The yield of the test is an important factor in weighing the cost of the screening program with its benefit. The yield is the amount of disease found in the population and is related to the prevalence of the disease. The higher the prevalence, the greater the yield.

Other considerations for the cost-benefit analysis of a screening program is how the benefit will be measured. The outcome can be measured by disease measurements such as the disease-specific death rate or case-fatality rate of screened group compared to the nonscreened group. The efficacy and effectiveness of the screening program are also important. The efficacy is whether the screening program works in real situations and whether it produces beneficial results. The effectiveness is whether the screening program reduces the total incidence in the population.

Example

Lead poisoning in children is a common and persistent public problem in the United States. The main source of lead exposure in urban areas was lead-based paint until regulations prohibited usage of lead-based paints for house and pottery. Lead can affect many organ systems. The main concern was for the adverse effects on cognitive development and behavior in children. Organized screening programs started in Chicago and other large cities in the 1960s. The New York City Bureau of Lead Poisoning Control established in 1970 is the largest lead poisoning control program in the United States. It is responsible for screening children, inspecting housing, and identifying lead-paint hazards. Screening occurs on high-risk children from 6 months to 2 years of age living in older houses or in poor neighborhoods. Children at that age are most likely to put objects in their mouths and eat foreign objects. Paint chips from old houses painted with lead paint are common objects.

Two screening methods are used: they are portable hematofluorometers used to measure zinc protoporphyrin from capillary blood samples and analysis of free erythrocyte protoporphyrin from a blood sample placed on filter paper. Follow-up diagnostic tests measure blood lead levels. Children that are identified as cases are treated and the exposure identified.

TERMS

Accuracy	How well the test detects the person who is really infected
Reliability	How repeatable the results are (precision)
Screening	The detection of diseased individuals who appear healthy in a population by the use of tests or other diagnostic methods.
Validity	How well the test measures what it is supposed to measure

Related Principles
Sensitivity
Specificity
Predictive value
Natural history of disease (Epidemiologic concepts of disease)
Prevention and control (Overview)

References
Cole, P., and Morrison, A.S. 1980. Basic issues in population screening for cancer. J. of Nat. Cancer Inst. 64: 1263-1272.

Daniel, K., Sedlis, M.H., Polk, L., et al. 1990. Childhood lead poisoning, New York City, 1988. In: CDC Surveillance Summaries, December, 1990. MMWR 39(No. SS-4): 1-7.

Eddy, D.M. 1980. Screening for cancer: theory, analysis, and design. Prentice-Hall, New Jersey.

Galen, R.S., Gambino, S.R. 1975. Beyond normality: the predictive value and efficiency of medical diagnoses. John Wiley & Sons, New York.

Morrison, A.S. 1985. Screening in chronic disease. Monographs in epidemiology and biostatistics. Vol 7. Oxford University Press, New York.

Needleman, H.L., Schell, A., Bellinger, D., et al. 1990. The long-term effects of exposure to low doses of lead in childhood: an 11-year follow-up report. N. Engl. J. Med. 322:83-88.

Thorner, R.M., and Remein, Q.R. 1961. Principles and procedures in the evaluation of screening for disease. U.S. Dept. of HEW, Public Health Monograph No. 67. USPHS Pub. No. 846. U.S Printing Office, Washington, D.C.

Sensitivity

The sensitivity of a test is the number of diseased individuals in a population who actually test positive on the test. It is the probability of correctly identifying a diseased individual by a specific test.

Explanation

Sensitivity is the ability of a screening or diagnostic test, by way of a positive result to detect a diseased individual. A person with a disease and a positive test is said to be a true positive. A person with a disease but a negative test is said to be a false negative. Sensitivity is the proportion of diseased individuals, expressed as a percentage, that are identified as diseased by the test. The more false negatives that occur, the less sensitive the test. If the test is less sensitive, it is less able to detect diseased individuals in a population.

The sensitivity can be calculated by the use of the familiar 2 × 2 table.

	DISEASE	
Test	**Yes**	**No**
Positive (Yes)	a	b
Negative (No)	c	d

a = true positives (those that test positive and are diseased) or

$$a/a + c$$

b = false positives (those that test positive and are not diseased) or

$$b/b + d$$

c = false negatives (those that test negative but are diseased) or

$$c/a + c$$

d = true negatives (those that test negative and are not diseased) or

$$d/b + d$$

So sensitivity is a/a + c or the number of true positives divided by the number of those who are diseased.

Few tests give strictly yes or no results. Usually a cut-off level is set to determine what result is considered positive and what result is considered negative. If a narrow cut-off level is determined for a positive result, then it is more likely for some test results to be considered negative when they are in fact positive. A narrow cut-off level makes a screening test less sensitive and allows more false negatives. The percentage of false negatives is the complement of sensitivity. If the cut-off level is more broad, then it is more likely for the test results to be considered positive even though the test may actually be negative. The screening test will be more sensitive but will also allow more false positives; that is, some healthy individuals will test positive. When determining the cut-off level for a positive test, it is important to evaluate whether it is easier to have more false positives or more false negatives.

Example

Although there is no evidence, the employers of a particular firm are worried about the radiation effects from job exposure causing a rise in breast cancer in the female employees. A mammography screening program is implemented in the workforce. The results of the first screening are:

	DISEASE	
Test	Yes	No
Positive	100	100
Negative	20	1000

Sensitivity = 100/120 or 83%

False neg = 20/120 or 17% or 1 − sensitivity = false negatives

$(1 - 0.83 = 0.17)$

The same example is used for the next two concepts to show how sensitivity, specificity, and predictive value are related with each other.

TERMS

False Negatives	The number of diseased individuals that test negative
False Positives	The number of healthy individuals that test positive
Sensitivity	The ability of a test, by a positive result, to detect a diseased individual in a population
True Negatives	The number of healthy individuals that test negative
True Positives	The number of diseased individuals that test positive

Related Principles

Specificity

Predictive value

Screening
Population medicine (Overview)

References

Galen, R.S., Gambino, S.R. 1975. Beyond normality: the predictive value and efficiency of medical diagnoses. John Wiley & Sons, New York.

Mausner, J.S., and Kramer, S. 1985. Mausner and Bahn, Epidemiology: an introductory text. W.B. Saunders Company. Philadelphia, Pennsylvania.

Roht, L.H., Selwyn B.J., Holguin, A.H., and Christensen, B.L. 1982. Principles of epidemiology: a self-teaching guide. Academic Press. Orlando, Florida

Specificity

The specificity of a test is the ability, by way of a negative result, to identify the number of healthy individuals. It is the probability of correctly identifying a healthy individual by a specific test. Specificity is inversely related to sensitivity.

Explanation

Specificity is the ability of the test to show a negative result on a healthy individual. It is the proportion of healthy individuals who show up negative on a screening or diagnostic test. A person without disease and a negative test is said to be a true negative. On the other hand, a person without disease but tests positive is said to be a false positive. The more false positives, the less specific the test. If a test is less specific, it is less likely to detect healthy individuals. The percentage of false positives is the complement of specificity. Like sensitivity, specificity can be calculated with a 2×2 table.

DISEASE

Test	Yes	No
Positive	a	b
Negative	c	d

a = true positives (those that test positive and are diseased) or

$$a/a + c$$

b = false positives (those that test positive and are not diseased) or

$$b/b + d$$

c = false negatives (those that test negative but are diseased) or

$$c/a + c$$

d = true negatives (those that test negative and are not diseased) or

$$d/b + d$$

Specificity is the number of true negatives divided by all the nondiseased or $d/b + d$.

Like sensitivity, specificity is affected by the cut-off level set for a diagnostic or screening test. The accuracy of a test is determined by the sensitivity and specificity. If the cut-off level is narrow, the test is highly specific but less sensitive. In other words, some test results are more likely to be considered negative when they are in fact positive (false negatives). If the cut-off level is more broad, the test will be less specific but more sensitive. In other words, some test results are more likely to be considered positive when in fact they are negative (false positives).

Since specificity and sensitivity are inversely related, it is important to decide what levels of specificity and sensitivity are needed for the particular disease being screened. A decision must be made as to whether it is more important to detect all of the diseased individuals, though some healthy individuals might test positive, or whether it is more important to make sure that healthy individuals test negative. For example, with a disease such as acquired immunodeficiency syndrome (AIDS), a false-positive test can cause tremendous suffering for the individual. AIDS patients suffer social stigma and the loss of health insurance, jobs, and friends. On the other hand, missing an individual infected with the human immunodeficiency virus (HIV) means that many other people may be exposed to a deadly disease.

One option to deciding between high sensitivity or high specificity is to do multiple testing. If more than one test is used at the same time, or in parallel, the sensitivity is increased. More than one test increases the chances of detecting a diseased individual. If more than one test is given in a series, then the specificity is increased; that is, another test is given to the positive individuals from the first test. More tests given after the first screening test eliminate the false positives.

Example (Same example as shown for sensitivity)

	DISEASE	
Test	Yes	No
Positive	100	100
Negative	20	1000

Specificity = 1000/1100 or 91%

False positives = 100/1100 or 9% or 1 – specificity = false positives

$$(1 - 0.91 = 0.09)$$

TERMS

Specificity	The ability to detect healthy individuals in a population with a particular test

Related Principles
Sensitivity
Predictive value
Screening
Population medicine (Overview)

References
Galen, R.S., and Gambino S.R. 1975. Beyond normality: the predictive value and efficiency of medical diagnoses. John Wiley & Sons, New York.

Mausner, J.S., and Kramer, S. 1985. Mausner and Bahn, Epidemiology: an introductory text. W.B. Saunders Company. Philadelphia, Pennsylvania.

Roht, L.H., Selwyn B.J., Holguin, A.H., and Christensen, B.L. 1982. Principles of epidemiology: a self-teaching guide. Academic Press. Orlando, Florida.

Predictive Value

The predictive value of a specific test is the ability to predict the absence or presence of a disease. The predictive value is affected by the prevalence of the disease in the population being tested. The higher the prevalence, the better the predictive value. The predictive value of a positive test is the most important clinically to health professionals.

Explanation

The predictive value of a test is the ability to determine the presence or absence of disease by that test. The predictive value of a positive test is the probability that a person with a positive test is really positive, and the predictive value of a negative test is the probability that a person with a negative test really is healthy.

The predictive value is related to the sensitivity and specificity of the test. The accuracy of the test, or sensitivity and specificity, determines its predictive value. The more accurate the test, the higher the predictive value. The more sensitive the test, the less likely a person with a negative test is diseased and the greater the predictive value of a negative test. Similarly, the more specific the test, the less likely an individual with a positive test is actually healthy, and the greater the predictive value of a positive test.

Unlike sensitivity or specificity, predictive values are affected by the prevalence of disease in the population. Regardless of the specificity of a test, if the prevalence of the disease is low in the population, then the predictive value of a positive test is low. The majority of the positives would be false positives. If the disease is common in the population, then it is much easier to detect a true case. The higher the prevalence, the more likely the positive test is predictive of the disease.

The predictive value of a positive test is more important clinically to the health professional. Detecting asymptomatic or subclinical individuals allows the physician an opportunity to treat the disease or at least control its progression. The predictive value is important in deciding about the cost/benefit of a screening program. If the predictive value is low such as 20%, then 80% of those testing positive will have to go through an expensive diagnostic work-up, though they are actually negative for a disease.

The predictive value of a positive test is the number of true positives divided by all test positives. The predictive value of a negative test is the number of true negatives divided by all test negatives. Sensitivity and specificity do not change directly with prevalence, but the predictive value does. With the 2×2 table, the sensitivity and specificity can be calculated from the prevalence in a population and predictive value; the predictive value can be calculated by the sensitivity, specificity, and prevalence of the disease in the population.

DISEASE

Test	Yes	No
Positive	a	b
Negative	c	d

a = true positives (those that test positive and are diseased) or

$$a/a + c$$

b = false positives (those that test positive and are not diseased) or

$$b/b + d$$

c = false negatives (those that test negative but are diseased) or

$$c/a + c$$

d = true negatives (those that test negative and are not diseased) or

$$d/b + d$$

Predictive value of positive test is $a/a + b$
Predictive value of negative test is $d/c + d$

Example

DISEASE

Test	Yes	No
Positive	100	100
Negative	20	1000

Predictive Value of Positive test = 100/200 = 0.50 or 50%
Predictive Value of Negative test = 1000/1020 = 0.98 or 98%

Sensitivity = 100/120 = 83%
Specificity = 1000/1100 = 91%

Now, let us assume that the prevalence of the disease increases in the population, then the 2 × 2 table looks like this:

DISEASE

Test	Yes	No
Positive	150	90
Negative	30	1010

Then the results are:
Predictive value of a Positive Test = 150/240 = 0.63 or 63%
Predictive value of a Negative Test = 1010/1040 = 0.97 or 97%

Sensitivity = 150/180 = 0.83 or 83%
Specificity = 1010/1100 = 0.91 or 91%

The specificity and sensitivity of the test do not change with prevalence; the predictive value does.

TERMS

Predictive Value	The ability of a screening or diagnostic test to predict the absence or presence of a disease in a population
Predictive Value of a Negative Test	The ability of a test to predict the absence of a disease
Predictive Value of a Positive Test	The ability of a test to predict the presence of a disease

Related Principles
Sensitivity
Specificity
Screening
Population medicine (Overview)

References
Galen, R.S., and Gambino, S.R. 1975. Beyond normality: the predictive
    value and efficiency of medical diagnoses. Wiley & Sons, New York.
Rogan, W.J., and Gladen, B. 1978. Estimating prevalence from the
    results of a screening test. Am. J. of Epidemiol. 107:71-76.
Vecchio, T.J. 1966. Predictive value of a single diagnostic test in a unse-
    lected populations. New. Engl. J. of Med. 271:1171-1173.

Surveillance: Study Questions

1. Explain the differences between active and passive surveillance systems and the advantages and disadvantages of both.
2. Give examples, other than mentioned in the text, of active and passive surveillance systems.
3. Suppose you want to add a reportable disease to the states' required list. What are the arguments for and against adding a specific disease to the list? What questions do you need to ask before establishing surveillance for a disease?
4. Why cannot screening programs be used in any population for a disease that you might be interested in?
5. What are the issues that need to be considered before implementing a screening program?
6. If the screening test costs $30 per person, is fairly accurate (65%), and has a yield of about 50%, would you consider a screening program? What if the yield was 84%? What if the accuracy was 97%?
7. Describe a disease where high sensitivity is the most important issue? Why?
8. Describe a disease where high specificity is the most important issue? Why?
9. What is the effect of low prevalence of a disease on the sensitivity, specificity, and predictive value of the screening test?
10. If you have low sensitivity, is there a high number of false positives or negatives?
11. If you have low specificity, is there a high number of false positives or negatives?

12. The prevalence of disease A is 2.0% in a population of 10,000 people that are being screened. The sensitivity is 50% and the specificity is 90%. Fill in the 2 × 2 table and calculate the percentage of false positives, negatives, and the predictive value of a positive and negative test.

DISEASE

Test	Positive	Negative
Positive	____	____
Negative	____	____

13. Assume the same situation as question 12, but the prevalence has changed from 2.0% to 5.0% in the population. The sensitivity is still 50% and the specificity is still 90%. Calculate the percentage of false positives and negatives, and the predictive value of a positive and negative test. What concept does this example demonstrate?

Index